Complications in
Cosmetic Dermatology
Crafting Cures

Complications in
Cosmetic Dermatology
Crafting Cures

Editor

Ganesh S Pai MD DVD

Former Director, Professor, and Head of Dermatology
Recipient of Professor KC Kandhari Lifetime Achievement Award (2016)
President, Dermacon 2015, Mangalore
National President, Indian Association of Dermatologists, Venereologists, and
Leprologists (2000)
Teaching Faculty in 5 Continent Congress, Dermatologic Aesthetic Surgery International
League, and International Master Course on Aesthetic Science

Foreword

Venkataram Mysore

JAYPEE *The Health Sciences Publisher*

New Delhi l London l Philadelphia l Panama

Jaypee Brothers Medical Publishers (P) Ltd

Headquarters

Jaypee Brothers Medical Publishers (P) Ltd
4838/24, Ansari Road, Daryaganj
New Delhi 110 002, India
Phone: +91-11-43574357
Fax: +91-11-43574314
Email: jaypee@jaypeebrothers.com

Overseas Offices

J.P. Medical Ltd
83 Victoria Street, London
SW1H 0HW (UK)
Phone: +44 20 3170 8910
Fax: +44 (0)20 3008 6180
Email: info@jpmedpub.com

Jaypee Medical Inc
325 Chestnul Street
Suite 412, Philadelphia, PA 19106, USA
Phone: +1 267-519-9789
Email: support@jpmedus.com

Jaypee-Highlights Medical Publishers Inc
City of Knowledge, Bld. 237, Clayton
Panama City, Panama
Phone: +1 507-301-0496
Fax: +1 507-301-0499
Email: cservice@jphmedical.com

Jaypee Brothers Medical Publishers (P) Ltd
17/1-B Babar Road, Block-B, Shaymali
Mohammadpur, Dhaka-1207
Bangladesh
Mobile: +08801912003485
Email: jaypeedhaka@gmail.com

Jaypee Brothers Medical Publishers (P) Ltd
Bhotahity, Kathmandu, Nepal
Phone: +977-9741283608
Email: kathmandu@jaypeebrothers.com

Website: www.jaypeebrothers.com
Website: www.jaypeedigital.com

Complications in Cosmetic Dermatology: Crafting Cures

First Edition: **2016**

ISBN: 978-93-85891-87-8

Printed at Replika Press Pvt. Ltd.

Dedicated to

My mother Shanta, who at the age of 94, is able to witness the publication of this book and feel proud of her son; to my late father Professor M Srinivas Pai, who instilled values and discipline in me

My children, Hema, a gynecologist, and Harsha, an ophthalmologist, who have grown to be young leaders in their specialties, and my son-in-law Prashant, an accomplished anesthetist

My three granddaughters, Neha, Deeksha, and Nilima, who have filled my world with joy and innocent chatter

My daughter-in-law, Anusha, who has shared the burden of scrutinizing and organizing the chapters with painstaking detail

Above all, my wife Lata, who has been through the ups and downs in my career.

Contributors

EDITOR

Ganesh S Pai MD DVD

Former Director, Professor, and Head of Dermatology
Recipient of Professor KC Kandhari Lifetime Achievement Award (2016)
President, Dermacon 2015, Mangalore
National President, Indian Association of Dermatologists, Venereologists, and
Leprologists (2000)
Teaching Faculty in 5 Continent Congress, Dermatologic Aesthetic Surgery International League, and
International Master Course on Aesthetic Science

CONTRIBUTING AUTHORS

Sanjeev J Aurangabadkar MD
Consultant Dermatologist
Department of Dermatology
Skin and Laser Clinic
Hyderabad, Telangana, India

Madura Chandraiah MD FRGUHS
Consultant Dermatologist
Department of Dermatology
Cutis Academy of Cutaneous
Sciences
Bengaluru, Karnataka, India

Rajetha Damisetty MD
Consultant Dermatologist
Department of Dermatology
Mohana Skin and Hair Clinic
Hyderabad, Telangana, India

Rajul Davda MD
Consultant Dermatologist
Department of Dermatology
Skin Secrets
Mumbai, Maharashtra, India

Sanjay Dubey MD
Consultant Dermatologist
Department of Dermatology
Maharshi Vitiligo Centre
Indore, Madhya Pradesh, India

Anil Ganjoo MD
Consultant Dermatologist
Department of Dermatology
Skinnovation Clinics
New Delhi, India

Shikhar Ganjoo MD
Assistant Professor
Department of Dermatology
and STD, SGT Medical College,
Hospital and Research Institute
Gurgaon, Haryana, India

Kiran Godse MD DVD FRCP
Professor, Department of
Dermatology, DY Patil Hospital
Mumbai, Maharashtra, India

K Narendra Kamath MD DVD
FAAD
Consultant Dermatologist
Department of Dermatology
Cutis Clinic
Mangalore, Karnataka, India

Vaishalee Kirane DVD DNB
Dermatologist and Trichologist
Skin and Hair Clinic
Pune, Maharashtra, India

Malavika Kohli MD
Medical Director
Department of Dermatology
Skin Secrets
Mumbai, Maharashtra, India

Amit Luthra MD
Consultant Dermatologist
Department of Dermatology
Ishira Skin Clinic
Delhi, India

Aditya Mahajan MD FCPS DDV
Consultant Dermatologist
Department of Dermatology
Dr Mahajan's Skin, Hair and
Laser Clinic
Mumbai, Maharashtra, India

Hema Mallya MS
Consultant Obstetrician and
Gynecologist
Department of Gynecology
Derma Care
Mangalore, Karnataka, India

Prashant Mallya MD
Anesthetist
Department of Anesthesia
Yenepoya Super Speciality
Hospital
Mangalore, Karnataka, India

Narmada Matang DVD
Consultant Dermatologist
Department of Dermatology
Neo Skin and Cosmetic Clinic
Mumbai, Maharashtra, India

Venkataram Mysore MD DNB
DipRCPath FRCP FISHRS
President, IADVL
Director, Venkat Charmalaya–
Center for Advanced Dermatology
Bengaluru, Karnataka, India

Umashankar Nagaraju MD
Consultant Dermatologist
Department of Dermatology
Dermavision
Bengaluru, Karnataka, India

Sudhir Nayak UK MD DDVL
Assistant Professor
Department of Dermatology,
Venereology, and Leprosy
Kasturba Medical College
Manipal, Karnataka, India

Anusha H Pai MD
Consultant Dermatologist
Department of Dermatology
Derma Care
Mangalore, Karnataka, India

Harsha S Pai MS
Consultant Ophthalmologist
Department of Ophthalmology
Alpha Laser and Surgical Centre
Mangalore, Karnataka, India

Vindhya A Pai MD
Dermatologist
Department of Dermatology
Kasturba Medical College and
Hospital
Mangalore, Karnataka, India

Sathish B Pai MD DVD
Professor and Head
Department of Dermatology,
Venereology, and Leprosy
Kasturba Medical College and
Hospital
Manipal, Karnataka, India

Narendra Patwardhan MD
DV DVD
Consultant Dermatologist
Shreeyash Hospital
Pune, Maharashtra, India

Pavan R Rangaraj MD
Consultant Dermatologist
Department of Dermatology
Cutis Academy of Cutaneous
Sciences
Bengaluru, Karnataka, India

Avitus JR Prasad MBBS DDVL
DM
Chief Laser Surgeon
SP Derma Center
Madurai, Tamil Nadu, India

Savitha AS MD DNB
Assistant Professor
Department of Dermatology
Sapthagiri Institute of Medical
Sciences
Bengaluru, Karnataka, India

Chaithra Shenoy MD
Consultant Dermatologist
Department of Dermatology
Cutis Academy of Cutaneous
Sciences
Bengaluru, Karnataka, India

Chandrashekar B Shivanna
MD DNB
Medical Director
Department of Dermatology
Cutis Academy of Cutaneous
Sciences
Bengaluru, Karnataka, India

Kuldeep Singh MD MSMcH
Senior Consultant
Department of Plastic,
Reconstructive and
Aesthetic Surgery
Indraprastha Apollo Hospitals
New Delhi, India

Simal Soin MD
Consultant Dermatologist
Department of Dermatology
Aayna Clinic
New Delhi, India

Dhepe N Vishwanath MD
FAAD Fellow ASDS ASLMS EADV
ISHRS IADVL ACSI
Medical Director
Department of Dermatology
Skin City
Mumbai, Maharashtra, India

Foreword

Dermatosurgery is usually a safe surgical practice, however complications do occur and are an important part of dermatosurgical practice. The adage "there cannot be a surgery without complications" holds true for dermatosurgery too. And in these days of consumer activism, complications have assumed a vital part of the practice. However, complications are also opportunities to learn—they teach humility and teach a surgeon to get wiser and better. They teach the surgeon how not to do surgery, and also when not to do surgery.

It is, therefore, refreshing to see a book on this subject—and who better than Dr Pai to author such a book? Dr Pai combines the old generation skills of empathy and clinical dermatological knowledge with new generation skill of procedural excellence and entrepreneurship. He was one of the first dermatologists to make the transition from arm chair dermatology to interventional dermatology, and, therefore, he has seen them all! He also has the necessary teaching experience and communication skills to author a book on such a vital subject.

The book fills a void and occupies a niche. The book has included complications of all procedures—esthetic, surgical, and laser. It is a great guide to the beginner as well as the experienced. The authors are all highly experienced dermatologists from all parts of India and the book is, therefore, a mine field of information. I have no doubt that this book will be greatly appreciated by all dermatosurgeons.

Venkataram Mysore MD DNB DipRCPath FRCP FISHRS
President, Indian Association of Dermatologists, Venereologists, and Leprologists
Director, Venkat Charmalaya – Center for Advanced Dermatology
Bengaluru, Karnataka, India

Preface

This book took over a year to complete and is unusual from other books on lasers and cosmetology. It guides aspiring dermatologists towards safe shores; errors of judgment made by authors early in their careers, mistakes by fellow professionals which ended up in our offices, and unpredictable outcomes that occurred despite best attention all features in this book.

The authors are leaders in their chapters and emphasis has been made on practical concepts. Tips guide us from cookbook to kitchen with useful suggestions; salvaging good end results from possible disasters have been demonstrated.

When you begin your long journey in the world of lasers and cosmetology, there will be headwinds and foggy windshields which will make the journey troublesome.

Keep this book in the co-driver seat to make your journey safe and comfortable. In this day of demanding patients, we have to walk a tight rope between adulation and their litiginous bent of mind.

It is the fervent hope of our authors that this book will steer your careers to success.

Ganesh S Pai

Acknowledgements

I would like to thank all the authors for their painstaking efforts to produce chapters which harped on management of complications. It was a difficult assignment as a lot of effort was required to sift through complications and chronicle the results. Only cosmetologists with a large patient base and a bedrock of dermatology experience could compile data for such chapters provided they would set apart time for the project.

I would like to thank Dr Anusha Pai, who sifted through all the written material, arranged the photographs, and scrutinized the references.

A thank you to my teachers and colleagues of yesteryears and my former postgraduates who are the next generation of leaders in our chosen field. Indeed some of them are contributors to the chapters.

A special thanks to Jaypee Brothers Medical Publishers (P) Ltd., New Delhi, for bringing out this valuable book, especially Dr Neeraj Choudhary, who was the epitome of politeness and understanding in every meeting and telephonic conversation.

My thanks to Miss Bhavyashree for methodically organizing the write-ups and communication.

Thanks to all our patients who have enriched our knowledge of laser applications and helped refine our techniques. And finally to our readers, the large numbers of dermatologists in the length and breadth of our land. I hope they find it useful and enthuse us to bring out the next edition in future.

Contents

Introduction

Ganesh S Pai

Two decades ago, lasers were a curiosity among our dermatologists. In the last decade, we had textbooks with chapters on lasers. In the recent past, we have access to books by Indian authors on lasers and cosmetology.

It was time to bring forth a book which taught the right parameters and the correct way to manage complications.

There is science in lasers. The entire effect of lasers occurs when a stream of photons penetrates tissue and is attracted to the target chromophore: melanocyte, water, or hemoglobin. There it is converted to heat. Satisfactory results would confine the energy to the target tissue. Bulk heating would extend to surrounding healthy tissue and cause scarring. Therefore, it is the experience of the dermatologist which will determine if the lesion is well-ablated or collateral damage has taken place.

A qualitative evaluation of the skin is important. A clinical examination is always to be done in a well-illuminated place. A wood's lamp examination can diagnose melasma and vitiligo. When fluroscence is used, epidermal pigment is highlighted.

Dermatoscopy must be used to distinguish melanoma from benign lesions. When in doubt, a biopsy followed by histopathological examination of tissue is mandatory. Photographic documentation of the skin condition is important to record for many reasons. It is useful for follow-up and presents evidence to the patient of the improvement after every session of the laser. It also protects the doctor against medicolegal cases, which are increasing in frequency. A high end camera and large storage disc space are necessary to store and display high resolution photographs.

A staff in the clinic must be trained in photography. Spending a couple of hours with a professional photographer can help to significantly improve the quality of the photographs. Chin rests and standard lighting eliminates variables in brightness and color contrast. Make-up must be removed prior to photography.

Fillers and botulinum toxin are frequent procedures in our clinics. Choice of fillers and their proper placement are important. Wrongly injected toxin can lead to ptosis of eyelid. Wrongly injected filler can lead to blood vessel damage and hematoma. Facial asymmetry is the result of overcorrection. Therefore, the cosmetologist must have a thorough knowledge of vascular and neural structures in the facial anatomy.

Learning the primary use of glycolic, salicylic, lactic, and phenol peels is the first step to successful peels. Glycolic peels can have unpredictable results and have to be neutralized on time. Salicylic peels coagulate tissue proteins and work best on inflamed acne. Newer peels come in combination and claim a variety of benefits for pigmentation and aging skin.

As we read the different chapters on lasers, it will be seen how tissues react to lasers. At 60°C, DNA coagulates and at 100°C ablative vaporization takes place. This occurs with carbon dioxide and erbium lasers. More heat leads to carbonization. Photomechanical destruction occurs when high laser energies in a short pulse cause rapid thermal expansion of the target chromophore. This occurs with Q-switched lasers in tattoos and vascular lesions in pulsed dye lasers.

Photochemical effects occur because of reactive oxygen species causing irreversible oxidation of cells. It is used in photodynamic therapy with long pulse duration and low irradiance.

The exposure time is the most important factor because this will impact the temperature in the tissue. Ultimately, with experience, we can manipulate the laser's power, spot size, and pulse duration. Over a period of time, we will learn to get the best out of our laser machine. This will lead to ideal results.

Complications in Q-switched Laser

Ganesh S Pai, Anusha H Pai

❏ INTRODUCTION

Q-switched neodymium-doped yttrium aluminum garnet (Nd:YAG; 1,064 nm) is a highly pigment selective laser which targets endogenous melanin and exogenous carbon particles while treating the pigmented lesions and tattoos, respectively. The wavelengths between 630 and 1,100 nm are well absorbed by melanin. The Q-switched Nd:YAG generates an immediate ash white color at the site of impact due to heat induced steam cavities in the melanosomes which cause scattering of the visible light, producing a white color. Laser exposure dose is not sufficient if the clinical ash white color is not visible. Q-switched lasers deposit energy in the pulses of nanosecond range.[1]

The pigmented lesions are differentiated into epidermal, dermal, and mixed lesions. Epidermal pigmented lesions include ephelides, lentigines, café au lait macules (CALMs), nevus spilus, and Becker's nevus. Q-switched ruby, alexandrite, and 532 nm work well for epidermal pigmented lesions. Shorter the wavelength of the light, more strongly it is picked up by the melanin.

Dermal pigmented lesions like melanocytic nevus, Nevus of Ota, and melasma can be treated by using Q-switched Nd:YAG 1,064 nm, Q-switched ruby, and Q-switched alexandrite laser.[2]

The number of sessions required to get rid of the lesion depends on its size and depth, and the type of laser being used. Laser sessions can range from 10 minutes to under an hour. Nevus of Ota, Ito, and CALMS can be removed in 5–10 treatments.[3]

All laser treatments are outpatient procedures with none to minimal downtime, so patients are free to return to normal daily activities after treatment.

❏ TATTOOS

The number of young people getting tattoos as well as getting rid of tattoos has increased. Tattoo parlors and tattoo removing clinics are springing up in every city. There is a tattoo renaissance in people of young age, social classes, and occupations. It is considered body art and it makes them feel unique and special. In the United States, there are interesting findings—the higher the number of tattoos or piercings, the higher the risk of drug use and criminal conduct.

❏ TATTOO COLOR AND PIGMENT

- Black: carbon (Indian ink), iron oxide
- Brown: ferric oxide
- Green: chromic oxide
- Blue: cobalt aluminate
- Purple: manganese
- Red: mercuric sulfate (cinnabar)
- Yellow: cadmium sulfide
- White: titanium oxide, zinc oxide
  - Red tattoo pigment causes most tattoo pigment-based reactions
  - Cadmium sulfide may be associated with photoallergic reactions.

Tattoos can be divided into amateur, professional, cosmetic, and traumatic categories.
- Amateur tattoos: they are deposited at various depths of the skin by steel needle using dyes like ash, India ink, or coal. They use less ink and placement is superficial, making them easier to remove (Figure 1)
- Professional tattoos: artists combine organic dyes and metallic elements which are deposited in the dermal layer using hollow needle. Ink is typically placed in the mid-dermis and requires more energy to achieve adequate treatment; they are difficult to remove

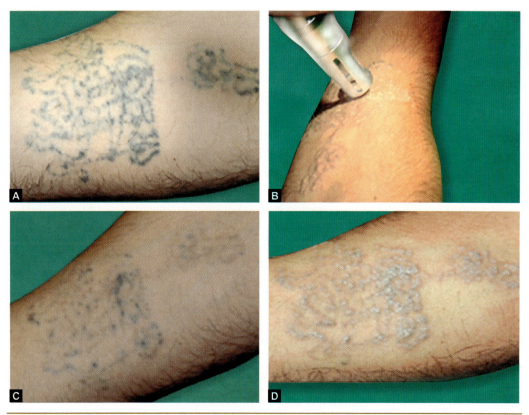

Figure 1: Amateur tattoo with Indian ink **A,** At visit; **B,** during procedure; **C,** immediately after procedure; **D,** after four sessions of laser.

Note: there is a small amount of pigment still left. Removal may be achieved by fractional carbon dioxide laser, followed by Q-switched 1,064 laser, 600 mJ, 4 mm spot size, 6 Hz, for each session and intervals of 2 months. With best efforts, full removal of pigment may not be possible.

- Cosmetic tattoos: skin colored tones are usually used in cosmetic tattoos
- Traumatic tattoos: nature of the trauma is important to know the depth at which the material is deposited.

Black and dark blue inks are best treated with Q-switched 1,064 nm wavelength. Red ink is best treated with Q-switched 532 nm wavelength.[4,5]

❑ LASER TATTOO REMOVAL

There is no single laser for perfect tattoo removal. Q-switched lasers fade most tattoos. About 75% clearance is realistic.[5]

After Q-switched laser, ferric oxide is reduced to ferrous oxide, explaining the occasional paradoxical darkening. The ferrous form is black and insoluble, which causes darkening of tattoo. Such tattoos can only be removed by an erbium YAG laser. A useful option is to do a test spot with the laser and to evaluate after one month (Figures 2 and 3).

Each color is absorbed by different wavelength of light, hence the more ink colors in the tattoo, the more difficult it is to remove. Removal of tattoo ink must be achieved with very short pulse width system in a nanosecond range (Figures 4 to 7).

In tattoos, the chromophores are exogenously placed ink within the macrophages or extracellularly throughout the dermis. Destruction of the pigment occurs through photoacoustic injury, which leads to rupture of the pigment containing cells which are phagocytosed by the dermal macrophages and lymphatic system. Superficially placed pigment containing cells are destroyed by the laser pulses, leading to sloughing of the epidermis and replacement with normal dermis (Figure 8).[6]

Multiple sessions are required to reduce the intensity of the tattoo. Whereas amateur tattoos may need 4 sessions at two month interval. The number of sessions for multicolored tattoos in unpredictable. Increasing fluence to shorter the treatment cycles may lead to burn injuries and permanent scarring. Patients must be counseled to be realistic and expect substantial fading of their tattoos (Figures 9 and 10).

Small spot sizes of 2 mm may lead to deep piercing injuries if the fluence is greater than 400 mJ; 3 and 4 mm apertures are the safest to work with depending on the width of the tattoos (Figure 11).

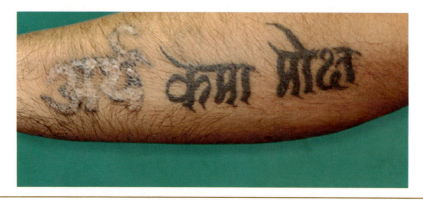

Figure 2: Patient from another center after undergoing multiple sessions of Q-switched laser.

Note: scarring caused by irregular fluence and irregular beam profile.

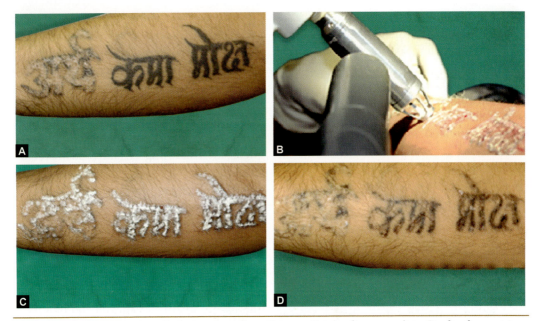

Figure 3: A, Before procedure; **B,** during procedure; **C,** immediately after procedure; **D,** after four sessions of Q-switched 1,064.

Note: change in color from black to brown due to change from ferric to ferrous form of tattoo ink. Further removal will need erbium laser ablation to prevent scarring (4 mm size, 800 mJ, 4 Hz).

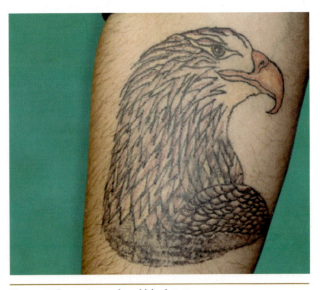

Figure 4: Extensive red and black tattoo.

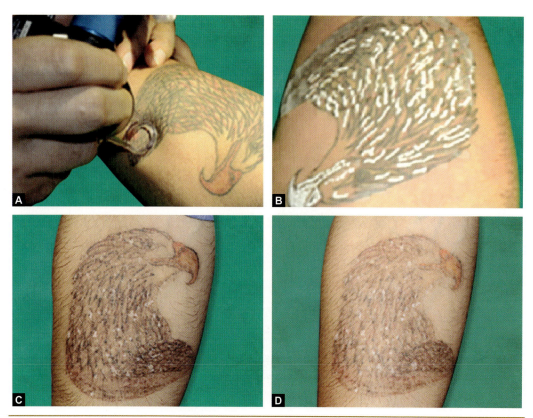

Figure 5: Fractional carbon dioxide density 5%. Size 10, energy 20 mJ used for initial pass, followed by three sessions of 1,064 Q-switched with 4 mm aperture at 2 months intervals over the entire tattoo. **A,** During procedure; **B,** immediately after; **C,** after 2nd session of helios zoom; **D,** after four sessions. From four sessions onwards, 532 nm is used to clear the red component.

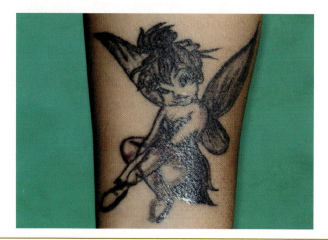

Figure 6: Predominantly black tattoo done to conceal scars caused by self-inflected injury.

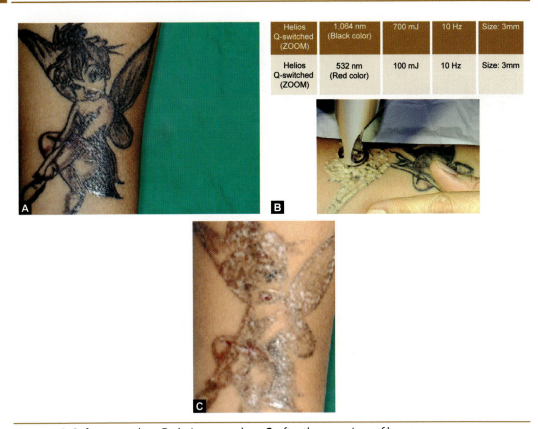

Helios Q-switched (ZOOM)	1,064 nm (Black color)	700 mJ	10 Hz	Size: 3mm
Helios Q-switched (ZOOM)	532 nm (Red color)	100 mJ	10 Hz	Size: 3mm

Figure 7: A, Before procedure; **B,** during procedure; **C,** after three sessions of laser.

Note: visibility of blade marks post three sessions of laser.

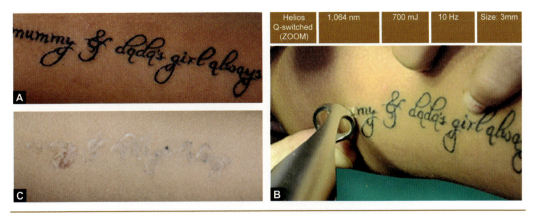

Helios Q-switched (ZOOM)	1,064 nm	700 mJ	10 Hz	Size: 3mm

Figure 8: Fresh tattoo removed 12 hours after tattoo insertion. **A,** Before procedure; **B,** during procedure; **C,** after one session. Removal is much easier as pigment is not amalgamated with dermal tissue.

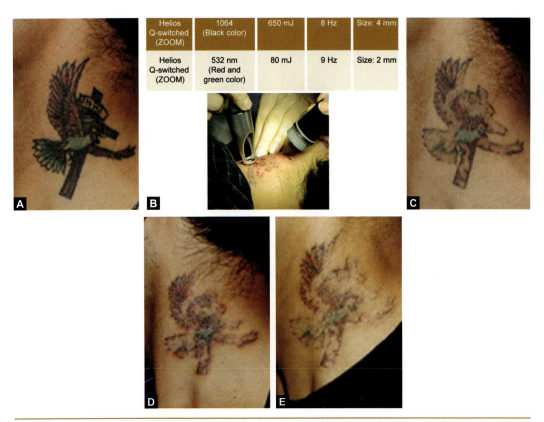

Helios Q-switched (ZOOM)	1064 (Black color)	650 mJ	8 Hz	Size: 4 mm
Helios Q-switched (ZOOM)	532 nm (Red and green color)	80 mJ	9 Hz	Size: 2 mm

Figure 9: Three color combination of blue, red, and green 532 and 1,064 nm used for different pigments. **A,** At visit; **B,** during procedure; **C,** 2nd session; **D,** 3rd session; **E,** after 3rd session.

Note: greater persistence of green color. Green is most difficult color to remove.

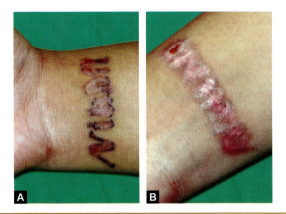

Figure 10: Tattoo with unusual demand from patient to ablate the name. **A,** Before procedure; **B,** after four sessions of laser. Q-switched 1,064 nm would remove pigment but leave behind etching of name. Fractional carbon dioxide (ultrapulse) done with higher power in the fourth session (first three sessions Q-switched-1,064 nm) helps diffuse the scarring.

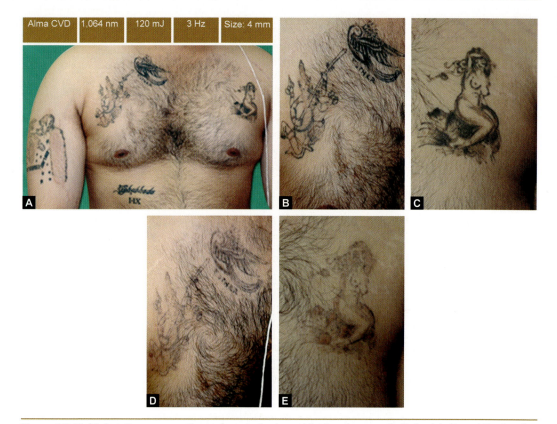

Figure 11: Multiple tattoos on a patient who required psychiatric reference. **A–C,** At visit; **D and E,** after five sessions of Q-switched laser.

❏ HISTORY TO BE NOTED IN A PATIENT WITH TATTOO

- Is it an amateur, professional, traumatic, cosmetic, or medical tattoo?
- Is it a fresh or an old tattoo?
- What colors of inks/dyes were used?
- Has the patient attempted to remove or alter the tattoo previously?
- Is the patient currently on retinoids?
- Is there a history of herpes infection in the proposed treatment area?
- Has the patient previously developed keloids after prior surgery or injury?
- Is it type VI Fitzpatrick skin type?

❏ TREATMENT OF PIGMENTED LESIONS

Lentigines and Freckles

The commonest form of lentigines is lentigo simplex. It is a benign, well circumscribed, small, brown lesion developing in childhood on both sun exposed and sun covered areas, mucocutaneous junctions, mucous membranes and nail beds. The skin creases are preserved. Histologically, there is increase in number of melanocytes at the dermoepidermal junction without focal proliferation or nest formation.[7] Neodymium-doped yttrium aluminum garnet 1,064 nm works well for the lentigines. Lentigines can be removed with one treatment (Figure 12).

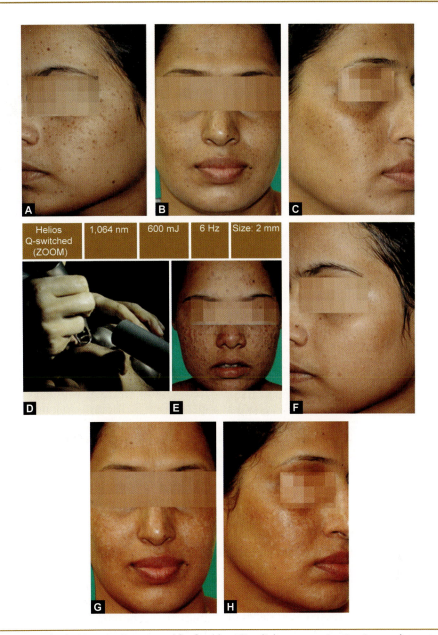

Figure 12: Q-switched 532 nm at 3 mm used for freckles. Wood's lamp examination is mandatory to choose the wavelength. **A–C,** Before procedure; **D,** during procedure; **E,** immediately after procedure; **F–H,** after 1 week of procedure. Those appearing more prominent are superficial and respond to 532 nm wavelength. Lentigines which appear less prominent are deeper and should be treated by 1,064 nm.

Freckles are small, poorly marginated, well circumscribed, pale brown macules present on the sun exposed areas in the fair complexioned individual. Histologically there is increased

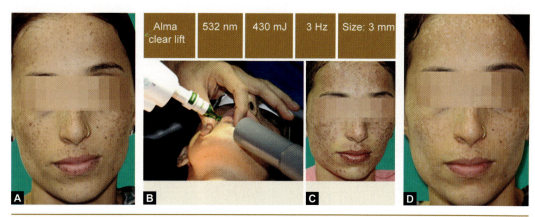

Figure 13: Extremely fair patients with light eyes and auburn hair often relapse after 12 weeks. Patients with freckles and dark hair have a permanent response. Notice the auburn hair. **A,** Before procedure; **B,** during procedure; **C,** immediately after procedure; **D,** after 45 days of laser.

production of melanin by the normal number of the melanocytes in genetically predisposed individuals. The pigment accentuates during wood's lamp examination. Neodymium-doped yttrium aluminum garnet 532 nm works well for the freckles (Figure 13).

It is advisable to perform test spots on the lentigines and freckles before treating the entire face. Test spots can be evaluated after 4–6 weeks. During the laser, there will be immediate whitening of the lesions. Patients should be advised about sun protection, postprocedure.

Café au Lait Macules

Café au lait macules (CALM) are discrete well circumscribed uniformly light-brown, round, or oval macules with serrated margins. It can occur as an isolated phenomenon or can be present as a marker of multisystemic disease, where they are usually large in size and are multiple. Histologically, there are increased number of melanosomes in the keratinocytes with a normal or slightly increased number of melanocytes in the basal layer.[8] Q-switched Nd:YAG, Q-switched ruby, and Q-switched alexandrite lasers can be used to treat CALMs. Multiple sessions may be required for the treatment. Postinflammatory

hyperpigmentation or hypopigmentation is common after the treatment of CALMs in the Indian skin.

Nevus Spilus

Nevus spilus is CALM with hyperpigmented speckles on it. The hyperpigmented speckles can be treated with Q-switched Nd:YAG but the CALM component can recur.

Becker's Nevus

Becker's nevus first appears in adolescence as an irregular hyperpigmented smooth macule on the shoulder, anterior chest, or scapular region. As the nevus grows over a period of time dark, thick hair appears on the surface. Histologically, there is variable degree of epidermal hyperplasia and increase in the number of basal melanocytes.[9] During the treatment of Becker's nevus, the hair should be treated first with the hair removal laser and then the pigment of the nevus should be targeted with the Q-switched Nd:YAG laser (Figure 14). There will be around 60–70% improvement at the end of the treatment. Minimum of four sessions are usually needed to reduce the pigment.

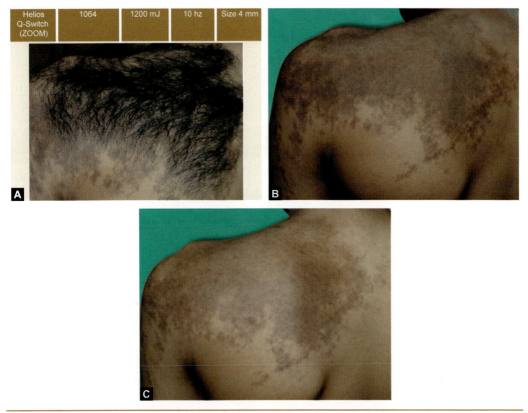

Figure 14: Laser treatment to remove hair is important before attempting removal of Becker's nevus at every session. **A,** Before procedure; **B,** after hair removal; **C,** after 1 year of procedure. Fractional carbon dioxide laser size 10, density 5%, 20 mJ, 300 Hz are done to break up the epidermis immediately followed by Q-switched 1,064 nm laser.

Acquired Melanocytic Nevus

Junctional, compound and intradermal nevus are the various types of the acquired melanocytic nevus. In junctional nevus, nests of the nevus cells are at the dermoepidermal junction. Q-switched 1,064 nm works well for its treatment. Compound and intradermal nevus will require a fractional CO_2 for ablating the fleshy part and then Q-switched 1,064 nm for targeting the pigment (Figures 15–18).

Melasma

Melasma is a common skin condition in Indian women. Various factors like sunlight, hormones, drugs, and genetic causes play a pivotal role in its occurrence. Melasma is a dynamic lesion which tends to recur even after treatment. The epidermal melasma is easier to treat than the dermal and mixed variants. Patients should be counseled about the outcome of the treatment before starting the treatment. The routine use of sunscreens should be explained to patients. Q-switched Nd:YAG and chemical peels are done at a gap two weeks. Three to four such sessions will be required to decrease the pigment by 50%. Triple combination creams can be given only for a limited period of time. Rebound hyperpigmentation can occur in a few patients (Figures 19 and 20).

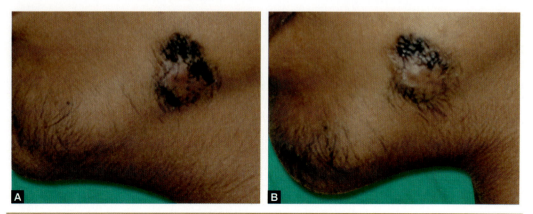

Figure 15: Teenage patient with nevus subjected to three sessions of fractional carbon dioxide followed immediately by Q-switched 1,064 nm at 4 mm aperture with energy of 1,200 mJ. **A,** Before; **B,** after 2 months. Notice the mild scarring and persistence of peripheral pigment. Patient may have been better off with excision by plastic surgery in the initial phase.

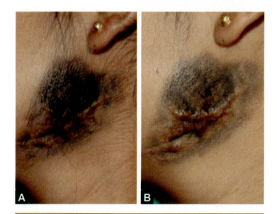

Figure 16: Similar case as figure 15. **A,** At visit; **B,** after 6 months of laser.

Note the hypertrophic scarring. Over a period of 6 months, scar will settle down. Further session of Q-switched laser can be used to ablate the pigment.

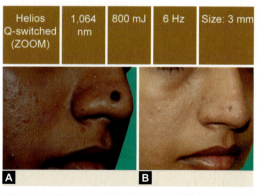

Helios Q-switched (ZOOM)	1,064 nm	800 mJ	6 Hz	Size: 3 mm

Figure 17: Mole removed by Q-switched 1,064 nm laser in single session. **A,** At visit; **B,** after 2 years of laser.

Note: slight depressed scar which is inevitable when there is a deeper component in the mole. Left alone, over a period of 6 months this scar base will fill-up making it a superficial scar.

Nevus of Ota

Nevus of Ota is unilateral patch of speckled blue-black, gray, or brown discoloration in the periorbital, forehead, malar region, and nose which develops after birth or during adolescence. The sclera is also involved at times. Q-switched Nd:YAG works well for the nevus of Ota. Five sessions will be required for the clearance of the lesion. The eye should be protected with a corneal shield while working around the periorbital region. The scleral component of the nevus cannot be treated (Figures 21–23).

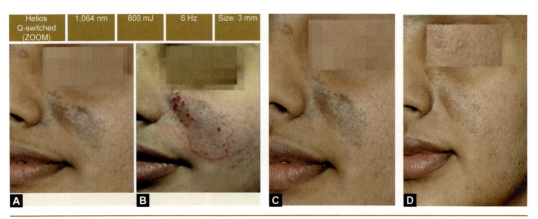

Figure 18: Four sessions done at once a month interval in such a patient. **A and C,** Before; **B,** immediately after procedure; **D,** after 6 months. A preliminary biopsy to rule out dysplastic nevus should be considered.

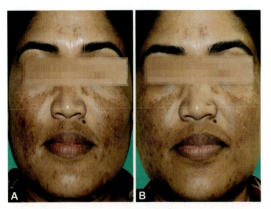

Figure 19: Patient after two sessions of fractional Q-switched 1,064 nm at 5 × 5 10 Hz, 500 mJ, and one session of fractional 532 nm at 4 × 4, 6 Hz, 50 mJ for melasma all at interval of 2 weeks. **A,** At visit; **B,** after 6 months of laser. Notice reasonable improvement in melasma and considerable improvement in acne.

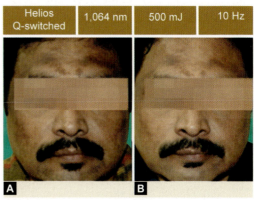

Figure 20: In 50-year-old male with chronic ultra-violet exposure after two sessions of fractional 1,064 nm Q-switched and fractional 532 nm Q-switched lasers (500 and 60 mJ, respectively) at intervals of 2 weeks alternatively. **A,** At visit; **B,** after 4 months of laser.

❑ HISTORY TO BE NOTED IN A PATIENT WITH A PIGMENTED LESION

- How long has the lesion been present?
- Has the biopsy of the lesion been performed?
- Has it grown, bled without injury, or developed symptoms like itching or changed color?

- Has the patient attempted to remove or alter the lesion previously? If so, how was this attempted?
- Is there a personal history of herpes infection in the treatment area?
- Has the patient previously developed keloids or abnormal scars after prior surgery or injury?
- Is it Fitzpatrick type VI skin? (Figures 24 and 25).

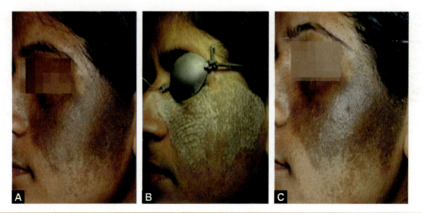

Figure 21: Patient with nevus of ota treated with two session of Q-switched 1,064 nm at 4 mm, 700 mJ, 10 Hz, size 3, over 6 months shows minimal improvement. **A,** At visit; **B,** immediately after procedure; **C,** 6 months after the laser. The patient did not come for further sessions. It is important to explain to the patient that visible improvement often starts after third session. Minimum of six sessions are required over a period of 12 months.

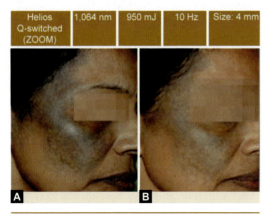

Figure 22: An extremely pigmented nevus of Ota. After six sessions of Q-switched 1,064 nm laser. **A,** Before procedure; **B,** after 1 year of laser. Notice the results are only moderate because the nevus of Ota was extremely pigmented to start with.

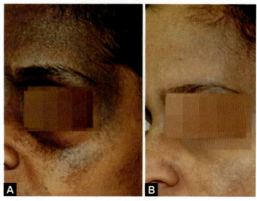

Figure 23: A very good result with six sessions of Q-switched laser. **A,** At visit; **B,** 2 years after the laser.

❏ PATIENT SELECTION FOR LASER

1. Thorough medical history including the history of allergy to anesthetics, current medical conditions, and medications should be asked for

2. Tendency for keloids, postinflammatory hypo- or hyperpigmentation and herpes simplex should be documented

3. Patients on isotretinoin should be treated after the stopping the medication for 3 month as there is a potential for increased scarring and delayed healing

4. Koebnerizing dermatoses such as lichen planus, psoriasis, and vitiligo are absolute contraindications for laser.

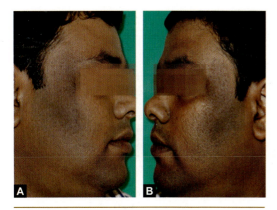

Figure 24: Obese individual with pseudoacanthosis nigricans. Q-switched lasers are ineffective. Fractional erbium/carbon dioxide laser leads to temporary improvement. Required is weight loss and lipid profile investigation.

❏ PATIENT PREPARATION FOR LASER

- Since removal of pigmented lesions and tattoos are painful, application of EMLA (combination of prilocaine and lidocaine), under occlusion at the treatment site is recommended
- Pretreatment photographs after informed consent from the patient should be taken
- Wavelength specific protective glasses or goggles should be worn by the patient, doctor, and the staff during the procedure. If the procedure is in and around the orbit then the metal corneal shield should be used
- Patients should be told to expect redness, swelling, tenderness, itching, dry skin, and black peppery specks, which may produce bronzed appearance in the days after the treatment. The specks or the bronzing are the clinical result of accumulations of melanin and so called microepidermal necrotic debris under intact stratum corneum and over laser induced dermal wounds. Various degrees of oozing, bleeding, bruising, crusting, and delayed peeling can be expected.[10]

Sunscreens are emphasized to limit the possible ultraviolet induced postinflammatory dyspigmentation.

❏ TREATMENT ALGORITHM

- Anesthesia
- Eye protection
- Determine test parameters
- Position handpiece 90° to skin surface
- Avoid stacking multiple pulses to same area as it causes thermal injury and scarring
- Pinpoint bleeders may occur. Edema will occur. Purpura is undesirable.

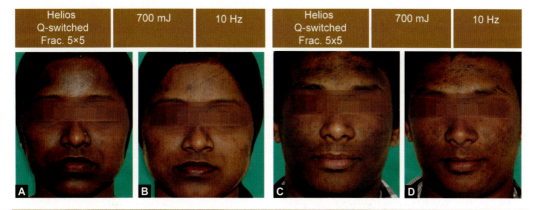

Figure 25: Individual with type VI skin: fractional Q-switched laser for photo facial 5 × 5 at 700 mJ generated postinflammatory hyperpigmentation. **A and C,** Before procedure; **B and D,** after procedure. 400 mJ would have been the ideal energy. Patient did not use prescribed sunscreens. This should be made mandatory.

❏ COMPLICATIONS RELATED TO Q-SWITCHED NEODYMIUM-DOPED YTTRIUM ALUMINIUM GARNET LASER

Postinflammatory hyperpigmentation or postinflammatory hypopigmentation.

It is the most common side effect encountered with the Q-switched Nd:YAG laser. The hyperpigmentation can be treated with the skin lightening creams and the hypopigmentation can be treated with phototherapy such as narrowband ultraviolet B. The pigmentary changes are usually temporary and will resolve with time. Patient with type V and VI skin may undergo depigmentation which may become permanent if patient has a history of vitiligo. Wavelengths of 532 and 1,064 nm should not be administered in the same sitting to a particular lesion as it may cause burn injuries.

Transient Erythema, Edema

The lesions appear edematous and erythematous postlaser, which lasts for a few hours to a day. There will be scab formation in the treatment of pigmented lesions which usually fall of at the end of one week. The patient is put on oral and topical antibiotic for healing.

Pain

The Q-switched laser when used to treat pigmented lesions is painful. Proper EMLA cream should be applied preoperatively. The lesion to be treated can also be cooled just before the laser. In hypersensitive patients, small areas can be injected with local anesthesia. Complications due to anesthesia rarely occurs.

Leukotrichia

The Q-switched Nd:YAG laser targets the melanin in the hair. The pigmented hair nearby the lesion treated with the laser turns white which patient complains as leukotrichia. The hair may regain its pigment naturally after a few days. Patient may be forewarned of possible permanent leukotrichia.

❏ COMPLICATIONS IN TATTOOS

Hypertrophic Scarring

When high parameters are used while treating the tattoos, there is always a risk of hypertrophic scarring. A careful history about hypertrophic scars and keloids should be taken before performing the procedure. In case there is hypertrophic scarring then it can be treated with triamcinolone injections.

Paradoxical Darkening of Tattoo Pigment

Tattoos with white and red inks are known to darken after the laser procedure. The white ink is made up of titanium dioxide which is converted to blue titanous ions. The darkening of the pigment is immediate and is permanent. It appears after the immediate whitening has faded off.

Tattoo Granuloma

Tattoo granulomas are common with the red colored tattoos. In the presence of granuloma, Nd:YAG laser is not advisable as it may worsen the allergic reaction. Ablative lasers like erbium and fractional CO_2 lasers are recommended to treat the granulomas and to remove the ink. The infective pathology should be ruled out before treating the granuloma (Figure 26).

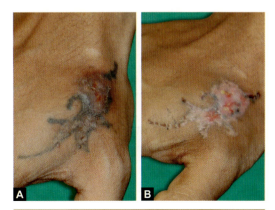

Figure 26: Allergic inflammatory response to red pigment in tattoo inserted 4 months prior to visit. **A,** At visit; **B,** after 1 week of laser.

Note: The ulceration. One week after fractional carbon dioxide for red pigment and 1,064 nm Q-switched for black pigment. Ablation of red tattoo is the first line of therapy. Subsequently, 532 nm Q-switched laser can be used for residual red pigment.

❑ CONCLUSION

Prevention of complications is an important step in management. History, physical, and pre-and postprocedural care contribute to prevention.

In order to prevent complications in Q-switched lasers, it is important to treat with moderate energy output in the first session. Spot sizes should also be 3 mm or larger to prevent deep penetration and scarring. The multicolored tattoos will need Q-switched laser which is specific ablation of tissue.

Good clinical acumen is required to rule out possible melanomas and basal cell carcinomas before attempting laser ablation of pigmented lesions.

❑ REFERENCES

1. Goldberg D, Dover JS, Alam M. Procedures in cosmetic dermatology series: Lasers and lights. Part 1 & 2; 2006.
2. Hruza GJ, Avram M. Lasers and lights: procedures in cosmetic dermatology series. 3rd ed. Saunders: Philadelphia, PA; 2012.
3. Lask GP, Glassberg E. Neodymium:Yttrium-aluminium-garnet laser for the treatment of benign cutaneous lesions. Clin Dermatol. 1995;13:81-6.
4. Adrian RM, Griffin L. Laser tattoo removal. Clin Plast Surg. 2000;27:181-92.
5. Grevelink JM, Duke D, van Leeuwen RL, Gonzalez E, DeCoste SD, Anderson RR. Laser treatment of tattoos in darkly pigmented patients; efficacy and side effects. J Am Acad Dermatol. 1996;34(4):653-6.
6. Kilmer SL, Anderson RR. Clinical use of Q-switched ruby and the Q switched Nd:YAG (1064 nm and 532 nm) laser for the treatment of tattoos. J Dermatol Surg Oncol. 1993;19(4):330-4.
7. Weedon D, Strutton G, editors. Lentigines, nevi and malignant melanoma. Skin pathology. 2nd ed. Edinburg: Churchill Livingstone. 2002. pp. 803-32.
8. Kim HR, Ha JM, Park MS, Lee Y, Seo YJ, Kim CD, et al. A low-fluence 1064-nm Q switched neodymium-doped yttrium aluminium garnet laser for the treatment of café au lait macules. J Am Acad Dermatol. 2015;73(3):477-483.
9. Danarti R, König A, Salhi A, Bittar M, Happle R. Becker's nevus syndrome revisited. J Am Acad Dermatol. 2004;51(6):965-9.
10. Manstein D, Herron GS, Sink RK, Tanner H, Anderson RR. Fractional photothermolysis: a new concept for cutaneous remodelling using microscopic patterns of thermal injury. Lasers Surg Med. 2004;34:426-38.

Protocols and Complications in Fractional Carbon Dioxide in the Management of Facial Scar

Dhepe N Vishwanath

❑ INTRODUCTION

Carbon dioxide (CO_2) laser has more thermal effect (coagulation) than evaporation (ablation) compared to erbium doped yttrium-aluminum-garnet (Er:YAG) laser, meaning more chances of complication like postinflammatory pigmentation, persistent erythema, and scarring. Carbon dioxide laser was an absolute contraindication for darker skin types until recently its fractional mode of beam delivery was introduced. High wattage devices delivering entire energy within very small fraction of time (UltraPulse) increased safety profile of CO_2 lasers to considerable extent (Box 1). Scars are collection of collagen that is abnormal in quality, quantity, and direction. Fractional columns of CO_2 laser induces partial denaturation of collagen inducing formation of new collagen fibers from surrounding tissue. Scars are less vascular and poor healer tissue. So, balancing injury pattern of laser to the healing potential of the tissue

is the key in avoiding complications of CO_2 lasers. This chapter discusses safe protocol of using fractional CO_2 laser in Indian skin mainly facial scars. Laser treatable scars and scar-like conditions have been mentioned in box 2.

❑ FRACTIONAL CARBON DIOXIDE LASER

Fractional lasers are the advancement in mode of energy delivery. In 2004, Manstein et al. introduced the concept of fractional photothermolysis.[1] Solid cylindrical beam of laser is fractionated into tiny microbeams. Instead of a wide column of bulk heating, discrete vertical columns of ablation and coagulations are created with normal tissue in between. This slight change in parameter will make a tremendous alteration in wound healing profile. Secondary intention healing is converted into primary intention healing which is faster, safer, and more restorative to normal anatomy.[2]

❑ SAFETY AND RISK PARAMETERS IN FRACTIONAL CARBON DIOXIDE LASER

Newer CO_2 fractional lasers allow variation of the thermal damage zones while others allow

> **Box 1: Golden triad of safety in fractional carbon dioxide laser**
> - UltraPulse profile on high wattage machine
> - Low density
> - High fluence

- Macular (pigmented or erythematous) scars
- Atrophic scars
  - Ice pick scars
  - Boxcar scars
    - Chickenpox scars
    - Acne scars
  - Rolling scars (valley scars)
  - Shallow atrophic scars
    - Stretchable
    - Nonstretchable
- Hypertrophic scars
  - Popular acne scars
  - Phymas
  - Surgical scars
  - Postaccidental scars
  - Postburn scars
- Contractures
  - Postburn contractures
- Keloids
- Stretch marks
  - Striae rubra
  - Striae nigra
  - Striae alba
- Morphea
- Fine wrinkles, lines, and solar elastosis

superficial and deeper penetration with a single scan.[1]

Width of Fractional Column

Width of fractional column should be minimal. There are two patterns of beams. Deep narrow fractional lasers (Deep FX on UltraPulse) have width of 100 μ and depth 1,000–2,000 μ. Second pattern is wide superficial with 1.1 mm (1,100 μ) width and 100 μ depth (Active FX on UltraPulse).

Ratio of Ablation to Coagulation

Carbon dioxide laser act by evaporation of water molecule in the target tissue. If energy is delivered in sufficiently short duration of time, cells get plumed along with vapors at temperature greater than 100°C and is called ablation. In this case of evaporation, there is no transfer of heat to deeper layer. If energy delivery is slower, tissue gets heated, coagulated, and sometimes charred and called lateral thermal damage that may cause risk of scarring and hyperpigmentation.

Ratio of Width to Depth of Microthermal Zone

For scar treatment, fractional laser beam should penetrate deeper without lateral thermal damage. Only UltraPulse beam profile and very high wattage can achieve this ablation column profile (Figure 1).

Pulse Structure

UltraPulse width of pulse duration is superior to superpulse mode (Figure 2). Continuous wave CO_2 lasers are no more used in cosmetic indications.

Fluence

Fluence is energy density, i.e. joules per square centimeter (J/cm^2). Highest possible fluence will reach maximum depth in one shot. In lower power devices, it is achieved by stacking of low fluence pulses that increases thermal component.

Density of Microthermal Zones per Square Centimeter

Safety of fractional laser depends upon normal tissue in between vertical laser beams. So higher the density, higher is risk of complications. In Indian skin, lowest possible density with highest possible fluence is the safety parameter. Higher density can be achieved by multiple passes of above safe, less

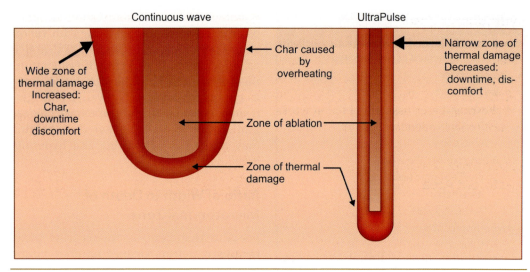

Figure 1: Ratio of depth to width of fractional column is key parameter of fractional laser safety.

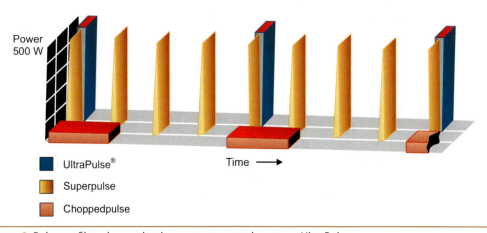

Figure 2: Pulse profiles: chopped pulse versus superpulse versus UltraPulse.

dense parameters. It is well established that postinflammatory hyperpigmentation (PIH) is proportional with how much basal cell layer is ablated. So multiple passes or higher density is associated with PIH.[5]

Repetition Rate or Stacking

In low power machines, high fluence is adjusted by stacking multiple pulses at the same spot. Additional stacking is highly risky in CO_2 laser in skin of color. Any fluence that is not able to raise tissue temperature to 100°C will induce coagulation of tissue protein and not ablation. Repeat pass on coagulated protein will end up charring. Char is carbon. Carbon has heat holding capacity till 600°C and called heat sink. This scenario at tissue level is worse than thermal cautery and will negate all benefits of lasers.

Hydration of Tissue

Safety in CO_2 laser is evaporation of tissue water and risk is heating of tissue water less than 100°C. Hydrated tissue improves evaporation and dry tissue leads to desiccation and charring. Laser tissue interaction works for safety only in adequately hydrated tissue.

Appendage Density in Treatment Area

Treatment area to be treated with fractional CO_2 laser is classified as "appendage rich" versus "appendage poor" instead of historical acral versus centrofacial classification. Appendage rich area, like face, has better healing and safety profile compared to appendage poor acral area. Atopic and ichthyotic skin is again appendage poor and a poor healer.

❏ WHICH PATIENTS WE SHOULD AVOID?

Literature mentions many scenarios as contraindications for use of CO_2 lasers. Those hold true mainly for surgical mode and continuous wave types of CO_2 lasers. Fractional mode and UltraPulse structure of pulse width has converted most of these absolute contraindications into relative ones.

- Recent tan is relative contraindication as it may cause PIH. A gap of at least 10 days from recent sun exposure is needed. A topical bleaching regimen is recommended by many but not proven to prevent PIH. Patient with outdoor lifestyle and lower socioeconomic status are often not aware that their level of sun exposure is high. Author has devised a test called "Sleeve test" to know the contrast between skin tone of covered skin and uncovered skin (Figure 3)
- Active herpes simplex or other infection on face

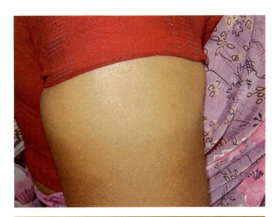

Figure 3: Sleeve test to judge level of tanning. Higher contrast indicates higher risk in the candidate.

- Severe active acne in treatment area: few lesions may not warrant postponing the treatment
- Appendage poor skin: acral areas are usually appendage poor. Facial skin, if dry and atopic, is considered appendage poor. Patient in figure 4 shows a case of melanocytic nevus treated with multiple passes of Active FX uneventfully. Similar protocol in similar lesion on acral area with poor appendage density ended up in hypertrophic and keloid formation that took several months of treatment to flatten (Figure 5)
- Pregnancy: though it is not an absolute contraindication, it is preferable to avoid these cases till the child birth for practical purposes
- Isotretinoin: concurrent use or use in past is described as a contraindication in various literature. In author's personal experience with more than 100 patients on isotretinoin, treated with fractional CO_2 laser, no adverse event like abnormal scarring or altered wound healing was observed in any case. However, patients are best advised not to be on isotretinoin till further scientific evidence is available

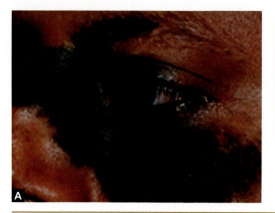
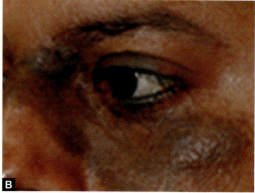

Figure 4: High level of safety in appendage rich skin: high fluence UltraPulse Active FX on face. **A,** Before; **B,** after.

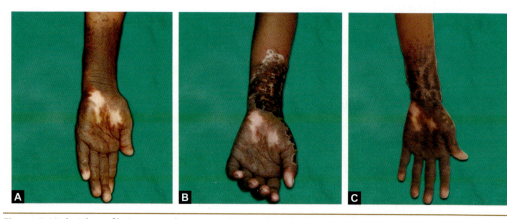

Figure 5: High risk profile in appendage poor skin resulting in hypertrophic scarring.

- Keloids: It is a relative contraindication. Treatment of keloids with fractional CO_2 laser when used in combination with fractional drug delivery of triamcinolone and 5-fluorouracil is found to be safe
- Resurfacing with fractional CO_2 laser is contraindicated in the presence of ectropion, prior blepharoplasty of the lower lid or significant lower lid laxity
- Unrealistic expectations: patients with body dysmorphophobia and unrealistic expectations should be avoided.

❑ TECHNIQUE AND PROTOCOLS FOR FACIAL ACNE SCARS (BOX 3)

Before Procedure

- Stop isotretinoin, if any, 2 weeks before the day of treatment
- Stop topical antiacne comedolytics two days before the treatment
- Check for recent suntan
- A bleaching regimen with double or triple combination is commonly practiced that does not guarantee avoidance of PIH

> **Box 3: Laser techniques in acne scar treatment**
> - Single tier technique: Deep FX or Active FX
> - Two tier technique: Total FX
> - Three tier technique: Total FX with scar shouldering
> - Four tier technique: Total FX with scar shouldering with high fluence Deep FX at base of the scar
>
> Note: All laser acne scar treatments should be combined with subcision on same day or on another day.

- Check for active herpes simplex labialis
- Preprocedure standardized photographs
- Anesthesia: Topical anesthesia with lidocaine and prilocaine (EMLA) cream under occlusion or nerve blocks in case of extensive scars
- Tumescent local anesthesia can be used on full face with or without nerve block while treating extensive scars or when multiple passes of laser is required. Face typically requires 100–300 mL of tumescent fluid and a higher concentration of lignocaine and adrenaline compared to tumescent fluid of liposuction
- Give a loading dose of amoxycillin and clavulanic acid antibiotic capsule and tablet lorazepam in case of extensive scars.

The Procedure

- Remove topical anesthesia on a smaller area. Clean the area with saline to remove cream remnant that may block optical penetration of laser light
- Keep smoke evacuator ready
- Protective eye wear for patient and operator. Face is prepared with surgical scrubbing
- Keep skin hydrated with wet gauze with normal saline
- Deep fractional laser is used as first pass with 10% overlap

- Superficial fractional laser: Active FX is used as last pass
- Shouldering is described under chicken-pox scars
- Reinforcement of anesthesia: if only topical anesthesia is used it wears off during first pass. A 1:5 diluted lignocaine solution can be massaged on laser treated area to reinforce numbness. This is adaptation of principle of "fractional drug delivery"
- Parameters used for acne scar are as follows:
  - Deep FX 20–35 mJ, 5% density, no stacking, two passes; second pass 45° to first pass
  - Active FX 150 mJ, density 3–4 on dial of 10, no stacking, up to 350 Hz.

Postprocedure

- Cold wet compress to reduce edema
- Healing serum or a plain white petroleum jelly to be applied on face frequently in a day in postoperative 3–4 days. It is widely believed that wet healing (closed bandage) is better than dry healing. White petroleum jelly is a nice adaptation of wet dressing
- No soap to wash face; use mild cleansers to wash face three times a day. Alternatively, water with little quantity of acetic acid (white vinegar) can be used for frequent face wash in first few days. Basic principle is maintaining pH of skin to acidic side prevents bacterial colonization. It should be kept on mind that soaps are mostly alkaline
- No topical antibiotic ointment is recommended as it may cause sensitization and future allergy to antibiotic molecule. Oral antibiotic like amoxycillin and clavulanic acid with nonsteroidal anti-inflammatory drugs twice daily for 3–5 days are given

- No steroid cream is recommended postoperatively to avoid sensitization. A single dose of prednisolone 0.5–1 mg/kg in two divided doses can be given (20 mg stat and 20 mg after 12 h)

- What to expect? Immediately after treatment face turns red. From the next day, small scabs start forming and face turns brown to black. These scabs usually fall on 5th–7th day. After scab falls, slight erythema is seen. At this stage, a moisturizer and sunscreen is added. A bleaching regimen with hydroquinone and with or without steroid is added after the 7th day of procedure

- Protocol: How many sessions and how frequently? With aggressive parameters, three sessions will yield 50–75% improvement in moderate to severe acne scars and more than 75% improvement if combined with subcision and scar shouldering.

❑ TECHNIQUE AND PROTOCOLS FOR CHICKENPOX SCARS

A three tier technique combining shouldering of scar border, subcision, and Deep FX of scar and surrounding area is employed. Scar shouldering is done with either 1 mm surgical tip of the CO_2 laser or in UltraPulse Active FX spot size 2 with fluence 150–200 mJ and 300 Hz. Base of scars is marked with surgical markers after surgical preparation of face. This 0.5–1 mm spot is moved on and around the edge of the deep chickenpox scar. The ablated tissue is cleared with wet gauze before second pass. A total of two to three passes of Active FX at edge of chickenpox scar are given. A pass with Deep FX at fluence 35–40 mJ is attempted at base of scar. The same technique can be used in deep rolling acne scars as well.

❑ TECHNIQUE AND PROTOCOLS FOR HYPERTROPHIC SCARS

Hypertrophic scars differ from keloids in one aspect that they do not grow beyond the limit of original injury. Hypertrophic scars have clumped bundles of nonpliable collagen arranged in haphazard pattern as against regular parallel arrangement of normal collagen. Aim of laser treatment to induce thermal injury to existing collagen leading to denaturalization that stimulates production of new collagen that is arranged in normal and more organized way. Postsurgical scars, postaccidental scars, and postburn hypertrophic scars are amenable to fractional CO_2 laser. Challenge in treating hypertrophic scar is reaching depth of 2–4 mm without extending lateral thermal damage. Most of low wattage CO_2 lasers achieves depth by means of pulse stacking at cost of lateral bulk heating. Only very high wattage device with UltraPulse configuration can maintain very high depth to width ratio.

It is worth remembering that scar is poorly vascularized and is a poor healer. Rox Anderson, opines that "Burn scars are caused due to injury that extends beyond healing capability by primary intention". Using another heat injury to heal the scar itself is a risky proposition. Ablation remaining fractional is the key factor and any aggressiveness in parameters will pose the advantage of fractional laser."

In SCAAR FX technology, depth can be achieved up to 4,000 μ (4 mm) without significant lateral thermal damage. SCAAR FX has made significant impact on outcome of hypertrophic scar laser treatment. Less density and very high power is the key here again. SCAAR FX at density of 3–5% and fluence of 60–120 mJ is used in scars with thickness of 2–4 mm. A 3% density with two or three passes in different directions to have more coverage than high density single pass.

Pre- and post-treatment protocol remains same except tumescent local anesthesia to topical anesthesia is preferred. Analgesia remains for hours after procedure in case of tumescent anesthesia. Three sessions is the minimum protocol while some patients may require more sessions depending upon thickness of scars and parameters used and adjuvant use of intralesional triamcinolone injections. Table 1 summarizes the typical efficacy of fractional CO_2 laser in burn scars at various intervals during treatment. The thickness and textural improvement is more than 75% in three sessions while color match to surrounding skin is less than 75%.[6]

❑ TECHNIQUE AND PROTOCOLS FOR KELOIDS

Keloids are different from hypertrophic scar. Keloids extend and infiltrate beyond the limits of original boundaries (Figure 6). There are many treatments commonly tried for keloids, none of them is uniformly effective. Now it is commonly believed that keloids are treated by combinations of various treatments. Fractional CO_2 lasers are used in combinations of pressure and intralesional triamcinolone with variable results. Deep narrow fractional CO_2 laser (SCAAR FX) to treatment protocol improves results significantly. Six to ten treatment sessions alternated or combined with intralesional injections and pressure gives impressive results.

❑ TECHNIQUE AND PROTOCOLS FOR MORPHEA

Morphea is an inflammatory skin condition leading to scarring changed in dermis and subcutaneous structure. Treatment combining anti-inflammatory treatments like excimer or ultraviolet B phototherapy, collagen remodeling therapy like fractional CO_2 laser and collagen stimulating therapy like platelet rich plasma results in significant improvement in early cases of morphea and moderate improvement in severe cases of morphea.

❑ COMPLICATIONS AND HOW TO HANDLE THEM

Common complications of fractional CO_2 laser (Table 2) and measures to handle them are discussed below.

Pain, Syncope

Carbon dioxide laser is painful and require anesthesia. Topical anesthesia is usually enough. For hypertrophic scars where deeper penetration of laser is expected, field block or tumescent anesthesia is required. Performing procedure in lying down position and painless anesthesia technique can eliminate chances of vasovagal syncope.

Postinflammatory Hyperpigmentation

This is the most common complication of CO_2 laser treatment in type IV–VI skin. Almost all

TABLE 1: Efficacy of fractional carbon dioxide in postburn scarring			
Point of assessment	Average VAS for scar thickness	VAS for surface flattening	VAS for color match
After one session	2.14	2.1	0
After two sessions	2.94	3.15	0
1 month after three sessions (the final assessment)	3.13	3.7	1.65
3 months after three sessions (the final assessment)	3.47	3.85	2.89

VAS, visual analog scale.

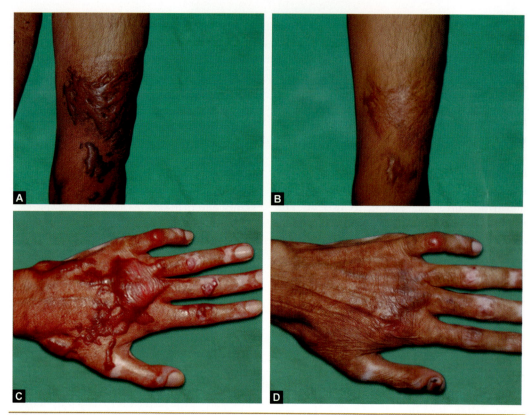

Figure 6: A case of hypertrophic keloidal scar of acid burn of 6–8 mm thickness, completely flattened with combination protocol. Similar results are expected in chest keloids.

TABLE 2: Common complications in fractional carbon dioxide laser		
Complications	**Frequency**	**Severity**
Pain	Common	–
Syncope	Common	–
Postinflammatory hyperpigmentation	Common	–
Postinflammatory hypopigmentation	Uncommon	Temporary
Erythema	Common	Temporary
Injury to deeper structure like panniculitis	Common with SCAAR FX	–
Infection	Uncommon	–
Reactivation of herpes simplex	Common	Fairly common in susceptible individuals
Reactivation of vitiligo	Uncommon	Fairly common in susceptible individuals
Reactivation of psoriasis	Uncommon	–
Reactivation of inflammatory disorders like lichen planus	Uncommon	–

Continued

Continued

TABLE 2: Common complications in fractional carbon dioxide laser		
Complications	**Frequency**	**Severity**
Contact dermatitis	Uncommon	–
Worsening of scar	Uncommon	Severe
Nonhealing ulcer	Common in contractures	Severe
Keloid formation	Uncommon	In susceptible individuals

patients will experience at least a transient phase of mild hyperpigmentation. Mild PIH should be considered as normal postprocedural sequel and not a complication. Darker patients, recent suntan, poor sun protection postoperatively, dry and appendage poor skin along with device parameters like non-UltraPulse profile, very high fluence, high density, pulse stacking will contribute to PIH. Preprocedural bleaching regimen using hydroquinone with and without steroids is recommended by many but with no evidence of prevention of PIH in scar treatment (Figure 7). Box 4 discusses measures to be taken to prevent or minimize PIH.

Postinflammatory Hypopigmentation and Erythema

It is an uncommon complication in Indian patients as against described commonly in literature for skin type V-VI patients (Figure 8). Immediately after falling of scabs skin shows erythema and hypopigmentation that slowly converts to skin color or PIH (Figure 9). Persistent erythema is rare and can be treated with vasoconstrictor gel or silicone gel application. Persistent erythema is better treated with vascular specific intense pulsed light (IPL) with filter at 540 or 570 mm. Newer duel filter IPL with filters at 550 and 600 nm (Dye VL on Harmony Alma) are very effective in managing persistent erythema.

Infection

Bacterial infections and fungal infections are uncommon after fractional lasers. An intense erythema and persistent burning in treated area is a sign of infection. A broad spectrum oral antibiotic cover is recommended when

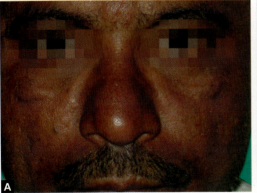
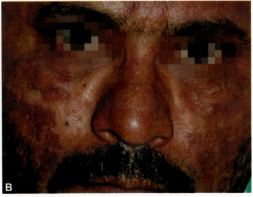

Figure 7: Postinflammatory hyperpigmentation in tanned patient.

Box 4: How to prevent or minimize postinflammatory hyperpigmentation?

- Golden triad of safety in fractional lasers
- Postoperative moist milieu with proper dressing
- A stat dose of prednisolone 20–40 mg, one tablet immediately and one after 12 h. Addition of triamcinolone in tumescent solution works in similar way
- Strict sun protection and start sunscreen from the 2nd day to be applied three hourly
- Bleaching regimen with 4% hydroquinone and mometasone from 2 days after scabs are fallen to be applied for 1 week daily in night then alternate daily for 2 weeks
- Avoid repeat treatment earlier than 6 weeks

full face or a larger area is treated. Topical antibiotics are discouraged as it may lead to sensitization and developing contact allergy to the antibiotic molecule. Washing hands with soap and water before touching the wound after treatment is recommended for both treating physician as well as patient.

Reactivation of Herpes Simplex Labialis

Treatment with fractional CO_2 laser on face may lead to reactivation of herpes simplex virus type 1 in susceptible individuals (Figure 10). Overall incidence is much less.

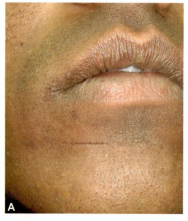
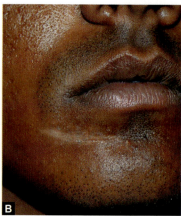

Figure 8: Postinflammatory hypopigmentation is common in tanned patients and in seborrheic areas.

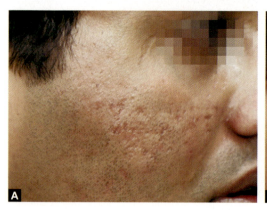
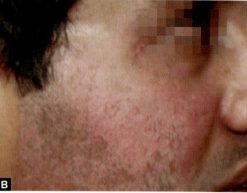

Figure 9: Erythema is common after fractional carbon dioxide laser. It is short-term in UltraPulse and long term in wider pulsed lasers.

This may lead to prolonged healing and undesired worsening of scars. A prophylaxis with 500 mg valacyclovir twice a day starting from a day prior to procedure continued till 3 days after is recommended in all the cases. At slightest suspicion of herpes infection, one should escalate the dose to full therapeutic dose, i.e., 1 g thrice a day.

Reactivation of Psoriasis

A case of burn scar was treated with fractional ablative laser and patient developed

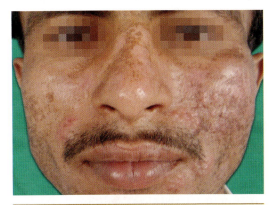

Figure 10: Reactivation of herpes simplex virus type I, though commonly mentioned in literature, is less common in practice.

abnormal scaling in treated area (Figure 11). It was diagnosed initially as infection and later as contact allergy and treated without improvement until similar lesions appeared on other areas of body. Within a week, patient evolved into generalized plaque psoriasis. It was a rare incidence of first attack of psoriasis triggered by fractional laser. Later prednisolone and methotrexate in appropriate dosages cleared the lesions completely.

Reactivation of Lichen Planus

Figure 12 shows a case of inactive, healed generalized lichen planus with postinflammatory pigmentation and scarring. Superficial wide fractional CO_2 laser (Active FX) was planned and performed at fluence of 125 mJ. This dose chosen in initial learning curve was clearly very aggressive and precipitated reactivation of lichen planus by Koebner's phenomenon. It was promptly treated with systemic and topical medical treatment.

Reactivation of Vitiligo

Resurfacing a patch of vitiligo is a common practice. However, an occasional patient may

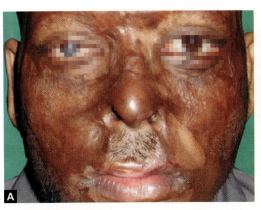
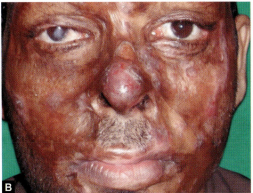

Figure 11: Precipitation of psoriasis after fractional ablative laser. In fact, this was first attack in this patient that took long to confirm the diagnosis till similar patches elsewhere appeared. Standard anti-psoriatic therapy resolved the lesions.

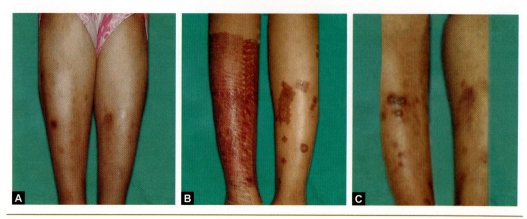

Figure 12: Reactivation of lichen planus after fractional laser. This case of quiescent lichen planus was treated for residual scars and pigment with fractional lasers, aggressive parameters resulted in Koebner phenomenon.

have Koebner's phenomenon and reactivate previously stable vitiligo. Figure 13 shows a case treated with fractional laser for acne scar precipitated into active vitiligo. This patient responded to topical tacrolimus, oral minipulse of steroids and twelve sessions of 308 nm excimer laser.

Contact Allergy

Contact allergic dermatitis due to topical antibiotic molecule or its sensitization leading to future contact allergy is common after fractional lasers. Fractional CO_2 laser creates channels into epidermis that remain patent for more than 48 hours. Entry of antibiotic molecule or its base into epidermis induce allergic response in previously sensitized individuals or induce sensitization making that individual prone for contact allergy in the future. Framycetin, mupirocin, and fusidic acid are common sensitizers. Avoiding topical antibiotics, giving oral antibiotic cover, using inert dressing medium like white petroleum jelly or other fragrance free moisture base, and using dilute white vinegar to maintain skin pH acidic will help preventing antibiotic sensitization.

Worsening of Scar

Very aggressive parameters of fractional CO_2 laser will eliminate all the advantages of fractional energy delivery and will render treatment as risky as traditional ablative CO_2 laser treatment, leading to scarring and hypertrophy. Restricting to golden triad of safety in parameters and safe patient selection parameters will help prevent this complication.

Damage to Deeper Structures

Initially, CO_2 laser, fractional, or traditional had limited penetration. With advent of narrow deep fractional mode (SCAAR FX) that has the capability to reach up to 4 mm, they had the potential to cause damage to deeper vital structure. There is a report of SCAAR FX causing panniculitis and draining necrosed fat over days through fractional channel. Traditionally, fractional lasers in patients previously injected

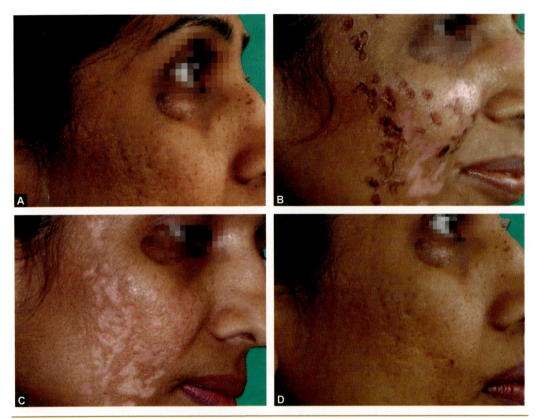

Figure 13: Reactivation of vitiligo after carbon dioxide laser in previously stable vitiligo case. Her depigmented patches responded to twelve sessions of excimer laser.

dermal fillers were considered safe.[7] Care should be taken while using newer deep narrow fractional CO_2. Therefore, adjusting parameters considering thickness of skin and underlying structures is the key for safety. Use of tumescent anesthesia in case of facial scars or burn scar has advantage of separating deeper vital structure away from skin.

Formation of New Keloid

It is rare but a possible complication. Low power device, aggressive parameters, unfavorable patient factors, and neck area of treatment are risk factors for developing keloid (Figures 14 and 15).

❏ CONCLUSION

Fractional way of energy delivery has made ablative CO_2 and Er:YAG lasers far safer and less ablative. Benefits of fractional lasers remain in fractional column of injury that is surrounded by normal tissue. Aggressiveness in any parameter will convert this into bulk heat injury leading to complications. High wattage machine, UltraPulse structure of pulse, and less density are key determinants of safety in fractional lasers.

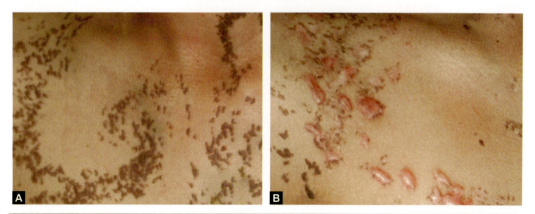

Figure 14: Formation of keloidal scar: low power carbon dioxide devices with more coagulation, failure to remove charred tissue in between passes, and inappropriate operative techniques are commonly implicated.

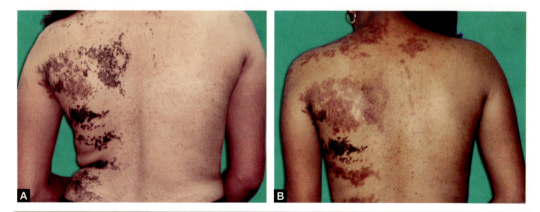

Figure 15: Erbium doped: yttrium-aluminum-garnet laser, UltraPulse carbon dioxide laser, removal of charred tissue in between passes yield safe results in similar case.

❏ REFERENCES

1. Hruza GJ, Avram M. Lasers and lights: procedures in cosmetic dermatology series. 3rd ed. Saunders: Philadelphia; 2012.
2. Manstein D, Herron GS, Sink RK. Fractional photothermolysis photothermolysis: a new concept for cutaneous remodeling using microscopic patterns of thermal injury. Lasers Surg Med. 2004;34:426-38.
3. Tierney EP, Kouba DJ, Hanke CW. Review of fractional photothermolysis: treatment indications and efficacy. Dermatol Surg. 2009;35(10):1445-61.
4. Dhepe NV. Scar reduction: principles and options. In: Lahiri K (Ed). Lasers in Dermatology. New Delhi: Jaypee Brothers Medical Publishers (P) Ltd; 2016.
5. Clementoni MT, Gilardino P, Muti GF, Beretta D, Schianchi R. Non-sequential fractional ultrapulsed CO_2 resurfacing of photoaged skin: preliminary clinical report. J Cosmet Laser Ther. 2007;9(4):218-25.
6. Dhepe NV, et al. Successful treatment of post burn scars with fractional CO2 laser in Indian skin. Lasers in Surgery and Medicine. Malden: Wiley-Blackwell; 2011.
7. Dhepe NV. Commentary on the Article,"Efficacy and safety of 10600-nm carbon dioxide fractional laser on facial skin with previous volume injections". J Cutan Aesthet Surg. 2013;6(1):33-4.

Complications in Erbium Lasers

Sathish B Pai, Sudhir Nayak UK

❏ INTRODUCTION

Cutaneous resurfacing using laser was initiated in the year 1994 with the advent of the ultrapulse carbon dioxide (CO_2) laser. The erbium-doped yttrium-aluminum-garnet (Er:YAG) laser was later introduced in view of the adverse effects and greater downtime noticed with the CO_2 laser. The multimode Er:YAG system—the tunable resurfacing laser—was thus developed.

Unlike the CO_2 laser, Er:YAG laser tends to bypass the plateau ablation characteristics and reduces the large residual necrotic areas noticed with CO_2 laser.[1] As the depth of Er:YAG's penetration is less than that of CO_2, the healing is rapid, but at the same time the dermal remodeling is considered to be also less.[2]

Erbium-doped yttrium-aluminum-garnet laser is ideal for superficial cutaneous ablation in view of the high absorption of laser beams by water. The wavelength of Er:YAG laser (2,940 nm) is closer to water (3,000 nm) in comparison to CO_2 laser (12,600 nm) and is thus absorbed 12–18% better than CO_2 laser by the superficial cutaneous tissue.[3-5] While depths of ablation comparable to CO_2 laser can be obtained with Er:YAG, it is often not preferred in view of the pinpoint bleed which occurs due to inadequate hemostasis.[4] The ablative properties of the Er:YAG has been attributed to the "microexplosions" of overheated water.[5]

The resurfacing properties of Er:YAG show more benefit than the collagen remodeling properties.[4] Even though Er:YAG laser shows good collagen remodeling properties, they are however slightly less than that achieved by CO_2 laser.[4] Laser parameters are decided by the laser system and indications. In fractionated Er:YAG or pixel Er:YAG, the laser beams are delivered as microbeams unlike in full field resurfacing where the entire laser spot is targeted. This delivery of microbeams produces microthermal zones (MTZ) with intervening areas of nonlased epithelial surfaces which lead to faster re-epithelialization.[5] Transepidermal elimination of dermal degenerated material also occur which is known as microscopic epidermal necrotic debris. Fractionated Er:YAG tends to produce superficial broad MTZ in comparison to CO_2 which produces deep narrow MTZs.

The tightening of the dermis and hemostatic effects of Er:YAG laser is considered to be inferior to that of CO_2 laser.[6] Improvement in skin tone and texture is often observed post laser (personal observation).

Various ablative fractional Er:YAG laser devices available include Pixel, ProFractional, StarLux 2940, Dermablate, and DermaSculpt.

❑ INDICATIONS[3]

- Photodamaged skin
- Atrophic scarring; e.g., acne scars, varicella scars
- Superficial wrinkles
- Hypertrophic scars and keloids
- Keratosis
- Epidermal nevi (Figure 1)
- Striae
- Verrucae
- Skin tags and anal tags
- Telangiectasia
- Spider veins
- Debulking benign tumors and cysts
- Actinic cheilitis
- Superficial skin lesions
- Diagnostic biopsies
- Decubitus ulcers
- Skin pores[7]
- Lichen planus pigmentosus (Figure 2)

❑ CONTRAINDICATIONS[3]

- Patients with unrealistic expectations
- Patients with body dysmorphophobia
- Active infection at site of resurfacing

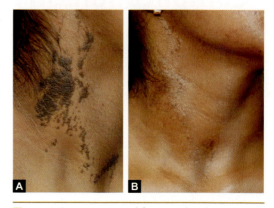

Figure 1: Patient required fractional carbon dioxide in the first sitting to debulk the tissue without scarring and fractional erbium subsequently after 2 months to smoothen out the lesions. Erbium 4 mm, 1,200 mJ, 4 Hz.

Courtesy: Derma-Care, Mangalore.

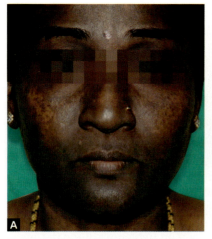 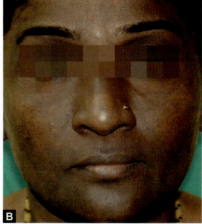

Figure 2: Lichen planus pigmentosus after 3 monthly sessions of fractional erbium laser. Gentle exfoliation of skin up to upper dermis. Fractional erbium long 7×7, 28.5 J/cm^2, 2 passes.

Note: Q-switched laser not used as it is ineffective.

Courtesy: Derma-Care, Mangalore.

- Hypersensitivity to topical anesthetic agents used (if used)
- Autoimmune connective tissue disease
- Photosensitizing medication
- Synthetic implants in treatment area[8]
- Malignancy in the treatment area
- Oral isotretinoin use in past 6 months
- Scleroderma
- Radiation therapy
- Botulinum toxin injection or Restylane® injections in the past 2 weeks.

❑ PROCEDURE

The authors used the Pixel 2940 system in the Harmony® platform for laser resurfacing. The laser beam is split into microbeams of diameter 150 µm. Two matrix sizes are available covering 11 × 11 mm². The 7 × 7 and 9 × 9 matrixes have 49 microbeams (28 mJ/P) and 81 microbeams (17 mJ/P), respectively. There are 3 operating modes each with possible increments of 100 mJ/P. The short pulse (100–600 mJ/P), medium (100–1,000 mJ/P), and long 100–1,400 mJ/P).[3]

The 2,940 nm Er:YAG module hand-piece is of 1 and 4 mm spot size with pulse repetition rate of 5 Hz and energy 200–1,200 mJ/P. There are three treatment modes available: gentle peel (1–29 µm depth penetration with increments of 1 µm), skin remodeling (10–330 µm depth in increments of 10 µm) and surgilight (fluence 100–1,200 mJ/P with increments of 100 mJ/P) (Figure 3). The pulse frequency in this mode is autoset to 5 Hz.[3]

- No pretreatment protocol is required usually,[1] but priming of skin for 4–6 weeks with topical retinoids/glycolic acid hastens the re-epithelialization process
- Informed written consent to be taken prior to the procedure
- Test patch on a small area (Figure 4) a week prior to the actual sitting is recommended so that the patient will be aware of what cutaneous changes can be expected on the skin till re-epithelialization and thus laser sitting can be adjusted as per any social events
- Concept of stacking: firing of laser shots repeatedly in the same grid without lifting

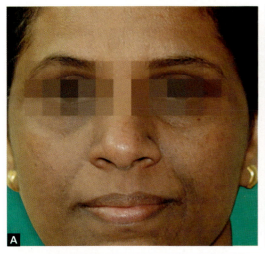
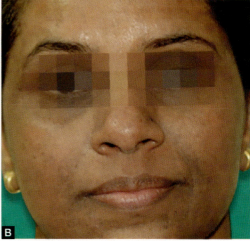

Figure 3: Facial with fractional erbium, 2 passes 7 × 7, 2,400 mJ.

Courtesy: Derma-Care, Mangalore.

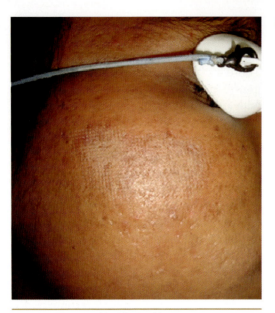

Figure 4: Test patch with pixel laser.

of the hand piece is known as stacking. In most lasers, stacking leads to an increase in the depth of ablation. However, consolidation of the desiccation tends to occur. Increase in the number of stacks leads to greater dermal changes. Initial passes lead to transmission of heat via the epidermis but once the epidermis is removed, there is a direct stimulation of the dermis. When 8 passes were passed, there is complete removal of the epidermis and frank thermal changes in the upper part of the papillary dermis, which has been confirmed by histological studies[9]

- Scanning fractionated Er:YAG hand-piece allow the delivery of microbeams of laser of same energy as full field energy that is in a scanned mode, thus enabling deeper ablation and higher fluences[5]

- In stamping delivery of fractionated Er:YAG, the laser beams are delivered in a single pulse. The laser beams are delivered as microbeams which are fractional parts of the total pulse energy.[5]

❏ STEPS

1. Remove any previously applied makeup or sunscreen
2. Wash face with water and neutral cleanser
3. Scoring of acne scars prior to each session is done to monitor the improvement
4. Pre- and postpictures in standard setting of position and lighting (to be taken after washing and drying of face, so as to have a better assessment of scars)
5. Topical anesthetic agents for fractionated Er:YAG laser procedures are not recommended as a routine.[3,8] However, it may be preferred in patients with low threshold of pain or anxiety. Also, it is necessary when ablative Er:YAG laser is used. If applied, then the anesthetic agent is applied under occlusion for about 30–60 minutes and is to be properly wiped out. The face is cleaned with normal saline and dried
6. Protective eye wear for both the patient (eye shields), operator, and other observers (goggles ≥6 and marked 2,940 nm) in the laser room is mandatory.
7. Matrix of 7 × 7 is preferred for aggressive resurfacing, while the 9 × 9 matrix is preferred for full passes and less aggressive resurfacing as in the periorbital area
8. Precool the area to be treated using external cold air, e.g., Zimmer®. If Zimmer® is not available, cold packs can be used. Care must be taken not to keep the Zimmer® too close to the surface, as distortion of skin surface may prevent appropriate laser hand-piece contact
9. The treatment area (usually the face) is treated in zones. The skin is held taut and the laser probe held at 90° to skin without any added pressure
10. Stacks are generally done over the scar areas before laser of the entire face is done, so that the scars do not get missed after the first pass

11. Usually around 6–8 stacks are done
12. The Er:YAG laser is then passed over the entire facial zone with minimal overlap in three directions, viz., horizontal, vertical, and diagonal
13. Feathering is done at the periphery of the lased area to merge with the normal skin, usually the jawline and hairline
14. The skin is gently wiped with wet saline gauze
15. Topical antibiotic cream is applied
16. Sunscreen is applied after about 15 minutes
17. The pixel tips and lenses are to be cleansed with clean cloth and warm water post-treatment as the tips are nondisposable
18. Sessions are repeated once in 2–4 weeks.

❏ PATIENT INSTRUCTIONS

- Avoid excessive sun exposure till re-epithelialization
- Use sunscreen post laser (Figure 5)
- Use soap free cleansers post laser
- Avoid exercises and hot water for 12 hours post laser
- Splash cold water or give cold compresses in case of any irritation or discomfort
- Avoid beauty parlor activities on the laser areas, α-hydroxy acids and retinoids for 7 days before and after laser sittings
- Contact sports and massages to be avoided until complete re-epithelialization
- Liberal use of noncomedogenic moisturizer to prevent dryness and flaking.

❏ POST-TREATMENT SEQUELAE

- Small white spots are seen on the surface of the skin immediately after firing the laser (Figure 6)
- This is replaced by erythema (Figure 7) and burning of the skin, which can last for few hours or one to two days
- On the third and fourth day, patient may notice mild edema or mild sunburn-like sensation
- Bronzing and flaking of the skin occurs on the fifth and sixth day (Figure 8).

❏ ADVERSE EFFECTS

Fractionated lasers often tend to have lesser adverse effects than ablative lasers. No serious

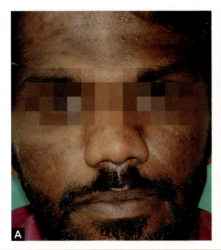
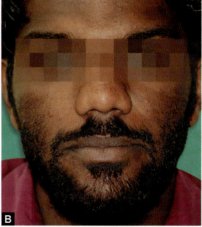

Figure 5: Fractional erbium in outdoor worker. Relative lack of improvement as he persisted sun exposure. Pixel long 7 × 7, 2,000 mJ.

Courtesy: Derma-Care, Mangalore.

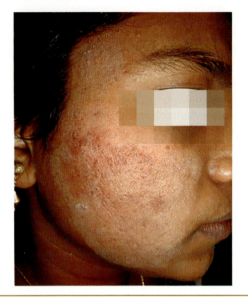

Figure 6: Small white spots seen immediately after treatment.

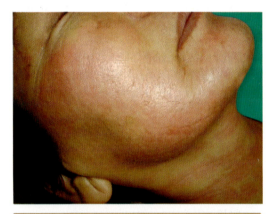

Figure 7: Erythema seen few hours after treatment.

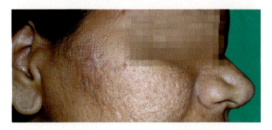

Figure 8: Bronzing and flaking of skin 5 days after laser treatment.

adverse effects are noted.[7] The fractionated Er:YAG laser is generally well tolerated with minimum to no side effects if done correctly. Discomfort and side effect incidence is higher in Er:YAG laser in the initial few days post laser whereas the same was more in long-term follow-up in CO_2 laser.[8]

Early detection of adverse effects is the main step in the treatment of adverse effects.

The possible adverse effects that one might encounter include:

- Discomfort and pain: usually transient and can occur in some during and immediate post laser. If persistent or occurring after few days, it is necessary to search for any foci of infection

- Prolonged erythema: post laser erythema tends to subside within 3–4 days, usually within 48 hours.[7] Any erythema seen after this is labelled as prolonged erythema. The usual causes for prolonged erythema include multiple stacks and excessive sun exposure post laser. This can be treated by strict use of photoprotection, especially sunscreens. Topical vitamin C has also demonstrated lowering the post laser erythema.[10] Occasionally, erythema can be sign of contact dermatitis

- Prolonged edema: usually post-treatment edema lasts for 1–3 days, usually subsides within 24 hours. Higher energies and excessive stacks are often reasons for prolonged edema. The post laser edema is often noticed more in the infraorbital region. The use of cold compresses and mild topical corticosteroids like fluticasone propionate will help in subsidence of this edema

- Dryness of skin: usually the post-treatment period is characterized by mild superficial crusting and dryness (Figure 9). The crusting and dryness tends to clear usually within 5 days post laser.[7] Aggressive treatment protocols may cause

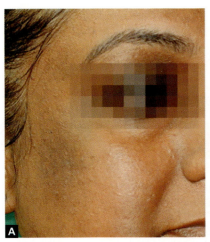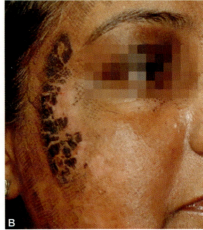

Figure 9: Fractional erbium full face photo facial with single pass, 7 × 7 long 2,400 mJ, 3 passes in the area of pseudoacanthosis nigricans. **A,** Before; **B,** after 3 days.

Note: scabbing after 1 week and eventually good result after 2 weeks. Lipid profile and lifestyle modification also essential.

Courtesy: Derma-Care, Mangalore.

this duration to be more. Frequent use of noncomedogenic moisturizers will help in improvement of the dryness (Figure 10)

- Pruritus: this is occasionally seen and is noticed when the erythema and edema have resolved. Oral antihistamines and emollients may be needed to prevent excoriations which are occasionally seen
- Increased sensitivity and rawness: this is usually due to the loss of epithelial surface post resurfacing. Emollients, sunscreens, and mild face cleansers help in alleviating the problem
- Post laser acne and milia: this is perhaps the commonest complaint from patients undergoing laser treatment.[7] The use of occlusive moisturizers, pilosebaceous unit injury, and aberrant follicular re-epithelialization are predisposing causes.[10] The use of noncomedogenic moisturizers post laser is advocated to prevent this. Patients with a strong history of acne tend to manifest earlier. Onset may be delayed in those who are not acne prone. Antiacne

medication like benzoyl peroxide, adapalene, or even oral antibiotics will be required to treat this. It is very important to inform patients to stop topical antiacne medication 3–7 days pre- and post-laser (depending on the antiacne preparation). The treatment of milia comprises of extraction with a needle

- Treatment of post-inflammatory hyper-pigmentation (PIH): patients with dark skin (Fitzpatrick skin type IV–VI) are predisposed to heal with hyper-pigmentation. The incidence of hyper-pigmentation at 6 months follow-up is statistically less in Er:YAG than in CO_2 laser.[8] Post-inflammatory hyperpigmentation often tends to resolve spontaneously. This can be best managed by use of strict photoprotection and demelanizing topical medications like hydroquinone, kojic acid, etc. Chemical peels may be considered to hasten the recovery
- Post-treatment hypopigmentation: like hyperpigmentation, post-treatment

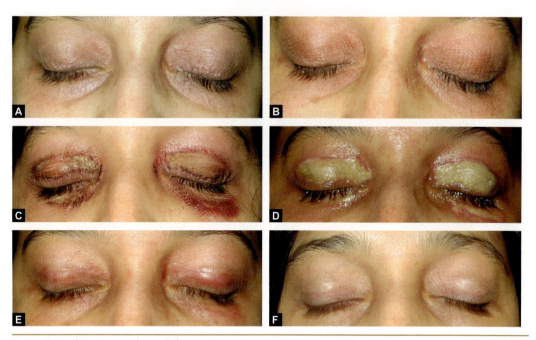

Figure 10: Showing vital need for continuous moisturizing post fractional erbium laser: **A,** At visit; **B,** immediately after fractional erbium for wrinkling of eyelids; **C,** after 1 week (patient did not apply prescribed ointment which lead to crusting); **D,** after 10 days (lasered area got infected); **E,** after 1 month (lesion healed with hypertrophic scarring); **F,** after 8 months (eventually good results).

Courtesy: Derma-Care, Mangalore.

hypopigmentation is seen; albeit in much rarity. Relative hypopigmentation (lightening of skin) may occur in areas lased in comparison to nonlased areas. True hypopigmentation is rare and is often delayed (6–12 months post laser). The hypopigmentation often tends to improve by itself. Rarely, it may persist. Use of sunscreen to prevent tanning in the surrounding skin is advocated

- Anesthetic complications: anesthetic toxicity is seen due to nonremoval of topical anesthetic agents prior to laser. The laser may help in enhancing the percutaneous absorption of unremoved topical anesthetics. This may manifest with perioral tingling, anxiety, palpitations, and light-headedness. Proper removal of topical anesthetic medicaments prior to

laser will prevent/minimize this. The use of lignocaine-tetracaine mixture of local anesthetics, especially for longer duration of occlusion, may cause erythema and edema in the areas of occlusion.[11] This is noticed immediately after removal of the occlusive tape and usually tends to subside within 24 hours. It is prudent to inform and show this to the patient prior to laser

- Blistering: this may be seen from days 1–3 post laser, especially when done for periorbital rhytides the incidence of this is more in Er:YAG than CO_2 laser[8]

- Herpes infection: eliciting a proper history of prior herpes labialis is a must before any laser sitting to prevent the occurrence of facial herpes simplex virus (HSV) infection. In case of any active HSV infection, it is prudent to defer the laser session till complete healing. Patients with previous history of recurrent herpes labialis will require prophylactic acyclovir/famciclovir/valacyclovir. Some dermatologists, however, prefer to prophylactically treat all patients with antiherpetic treatment. Antivirals, if started, should be given one day prior to the treatment and continued for a duration of 5–7 days. Herpetic infection post laser do not manifest with intact vesicles. Rather the development of superficial erosions especially if grouped should be considered as an indicator of HSV infection and antiviral agents started immediately. Polymerase chain reaction testing is recommended. Further laser sessions should be done under antiviral prophylaxis

- Bacterial infection: this is a rare complication and manifests as spots of erythema and crusts, fever, and increase oozing. The use of good hygiene like soap-free cleansers will prevent this complication. Short courses of topical or systemic antibiotics will be needed. Prophylactic antibiotics may be considered in immunosuppressed, patients with valvular heart disease[10]
- Fungal infection: cutaneous candidiasis is rarely reported after fractional lasers and is seen 7–14 days post laser.[10] Oral antifungal therapy is needed
- Scar: scar formation is a very rare complication post Er:YAG laser. This is often seen when laser is done either periorbital, mandibular, or in the neck areas.[10] Post laser infection, overzealous use of high energies, excessive overlapping passes, oral isotretinoin, keloidal tendencies, and decreased pilosebaeous units in the neck are postulated causes for scarring. Persistent erythema can be an early indicator for formation of scar in the future. The use of silicone gels, super-potent topical corticosteroids, intralesional corticosteroids, or even ablative resurfacing/pulse dye lasers may be needed

- Post laser purpura: often noticed around the periorbital area. The laxity of skin, rubbing/scratching post laser, and use of nonsteroidal anti-inflammatory or blood thinning drugs are postulated causes of purpura. The incidence of pinpoint bruising is comparatively more with Er:YAG laser than CO_2 laser in view of the lesser hemostatic properties of Er:YAG than CO_2[6]
- Contact dermatitis: allergic and irritant contact dermatitis are rare complications post laser. The denuded epithelial surface allows the easy percutaneous use of allergens as well increases the susceptibility to irritants. Topical applications often used post laser are possible causes of dermatitis. Stop all topical medicaments. History of any over the counter preparation use must also be enquired. Mild nonirritant face washes like cetyl alcohol to be used. Mild to mid potent topical steroids like fluticasone propionate ointment for 3–7 days will help in subsidence of dermatitis. Oral antihistamines may be considered. Patch testing with Indian standard series may be considered in patients with recurrent allergic contact dermatitis
- Superficial burns: this occurs due to improper contact of the hand-piece and is often seen along the contours of the body like jawline
- Recall phenomenon: this is the transient recurrence of erythema after subsidence of the initial erythema on taking hot showers or direct sunlight.[10]

❏ CONCLUSION

Complications in Er:YAG lasers are uncommon and usually easily preventable.

Awareness of precautionary and preventive measures are very important. It is essential to stress the patients about the need to use sunscreens and moisturizers, and following skin care regimen as instructed. Early diagnosis and treatment of complications prevent long-term sequelae.

❏ REFERENCES

1. Goldman MP. CO_2 laser resurfacing: Confluent and fractionated. In: Draelos ZD, editor. Cosmetic dermatology products and procedures. New Delhi: Wiley-Blackwell; 2010. pp. 393-408.
2. Tahiliani ST, Rais S. Management of acne scars. In: Sacchidanand S, Oberrai C, Inamadar AC, editors. IADVL textbook of dermatology. 4th ed. Mumbai: Bhalani Publishing House; 2015. pp. 2471-2.
3. Harmony® Multi-application Multi-technologyplatform Operator's manual. Israel: Alma Lasers Ltd; 2007.
4. Alster TS. Cutaneous resurfacing with Er:Yag lasers. Dermatol Surg. 2000;26:73-5.
5. Nemes K, Diaci J, Ahcan U, Marini L, Lukac M. Dependence of skin ablation depths on Er:YAG laser fluence. Journal of the Laser and Health Academy. 2014;1:7-13
6. Jung KE, Jung KH, Park YM, Lee JY, Kim TY, Kim HO, et al. A split-face comparison of ablative fractional lasers (CO_2 and Er:Yag) in Asian patients; postprocedure erythema, pain and patient's satisfaction. J Cosmet Laser Ther. 2013;15:70-3.
7. Karsai S, Czarnecka A, Jünger M, Raulin C. Ablative fractional lasers (CO_2 and Er:Yag): A randomized controlled double blind split face trial of the treatment of peri orbital rhytides. Lasers Surg Med. 2010;42:160-7.
8. Trelles MA, Vélez M, Mordon S. Correlation of histological findings of single session Er:YAG skin fractional resurfacing with various passes and energies and the possible clinical implications. Lasers Surg Med. 2008;40:171-7.
9. Metelitsa AI, Alster TS. Fractionated laser skin resurfacing treatment complications: a review. Dermatol Surg. 2010; 36:299-306.
10. Nirmal B, Pai SB, Sripathi H, Rao R, Prabhu S, Kudur MH, et al. Efficacy and safety of Erbium-doped Yttrium Aluminium Garnet fractional resurfacing laser for treatment of facial acne scars. Indian J Dermatol Venereol Leprol. 2013;79:193-8.
11. Sudhir Nayak UK, Sripathi H. Papular eruption secondary to prolonged application to tetracaine-lidocaine cream. J Pakistan Assoc Dermatol. 2013;23:245-6.

Vascular Lasers

Chandrashekar B Shivanna, Madura Chandraiah, Pavan R Rangaraj, Chaithra Shenoy

❑ INTRODUCTION

Cutaneous vascular lesions pose a great challenge to dermatologists. The lesions can range from superficial cherry angiomas to deeper hemangiomas and malformations to some abnormal leg veins. When choosing the ideal device to treat a specific lesion, the depth of the intended target matters greatly. An ideal laser with optimal parameters is chosen to expect beneficial results. Treatment of the same with optimal laser parameters is always rewarding. The initial treatment of vascular lesions with ruby and carbon dioxide lasers in 1960s was associated with a whole lot of side effects.

The new era in laser medicine began in 1983 with the concept of selective photothermolysis (SPT) introduced by Anderson and Parish.[1] The principle states that lasers or light energy produce selective heating and destruction of a targeted skin lesion which is chromophore specific, such as a blood vessel, without damaging nearby structures. Selective SPT first applied to port-wine stain (PWS) and vascular lesions were the first test cases for SPT.[1] Pulsed dye laser (PDL) was the first laser to show the selectivity for chromophore was practical.

❑ CLASSIFICATION OF VASCULAR LASER

The available vascular lasers produced excellent clinical efficacy with less scarring even after multiple repetitive treatments. A large number of lasers (ranging from 532 to 1,064 nm) and intense noncoherent pulsed light devices are now available for the treatment of vascular lesions. Pulsed dye laser, potassium titanyl phosphate (KTP), alexandrite laser, diode laser, and neodymium:yttrium-aluminum-garnet (Nd:YAG) lasers, as well as intense pulsed light (IPL) are being applied in the treatment of cutaneous vascular lesions. The laser surgeon should have complete understanding of the basics of lasers, intended target and of the device being employed for the procedure (Box 1 and Table 1).

Oxyhemoglobin (HbO_2) is the chromophore for vascular lasers. In order to target vascular lesions, the wavelength of light chosen must be preferentially absorbed by blood vessels. Vascular laser exploit selective absorption peak of HbO_2 by 70% and remaining by deoxyhemoglobin and methemoglobin. Oxyhemoglobin has three major absorption peaks at 418, 542, and 577 nm. Optimal absorption is within 577–600 nm range.[4,5]

> **Box 1: Vascular laser classification[2,3]**
>
> **Hemoglobin—selective laser**
> - Green yellow light sources
> - Long wave length lasers
> - Near infrared radiation lasers
>
> **Hemoglobin—nonselective lasers**
> - PDL (585/590/595/600 nm), KTP (532 nm)
> - Diode (800 nm), alexandrite (755 nm)
> - Diode (940 nm), Nd:YAG (1,064 nm)
> - Carbon dioxide laser (10,600 nm), Er:YAG (2,940 nm)
>
> PDL, pulsed dye laser; KTP, potassium titanyl phosphate; Nd:YAG, neodymium:yttrium-aluminum-garnet; Er:YAG, erbium: yttrium-aluminum-garnet.

TABLE 1: Types of lasers used for vascular lesions[3]

Laser/Light source	Wavelength (nm)	Pulse duration (ms)
Pulsed potassium titanyl phosphate	532	1–200
Pulsed dye laser	585	0.45
Long-pulsed dye	585, 590, 595, 600	1.5–40
Long-pulsed alexandrite	755	3–20
Diodes	800, 810, 940	1–250
Long-pulsed Nd:YAG	1,064	1–100
Intense-pulsed light source	515–1,200	0.5–30

Nd:YAG, neodymium:yttrium-aluminum-garnet.

❑ PARAMETERS FOR OPTIMAL OUTCOME

Wavelength: it is the first important factor, choosing the appropriate wavelength involves selecting a wavelength with enough penetration depth. Shorter wavelengths of 532, 585, and 595 nm target superficial lesions. Longer wavelength like 755, 810, and 1,064 nm can target both superficial and deeper pathology. Always remember the competing chromophore in the epidermis and appendages is melanin. Sufficient fluence is required for irreversible damage of the target vessel. Increase in fluence can increase the risk of damage to epidermis. Cooling is must to prevent epidermal damage. The lasers 755, 800, and 1,064 nm will have less interaction with melanin because of deeper penetration.

Spot size: it is the second important factor for both degree of coverage and depth of effective treatment. Bigger spots go deeper and also results in faster treatment. The ratio of dermal to epidermal damage increases as the spot size increases. Treatment fluences are, therefore, decreased with larger spots compared to smaller spot sizes. The rule being larger the spot size deeper the penetration and lower the fluence, vice versa is true for smaller spot size. When in doubt, smaller spot sizes are recommended, with manipulation of the fluence to achieve the desired energy at the target level (Table 2).[6,7]

Pulse durations: the third factor influencing laser outcome is pulse duration, it depends on size of the intended target. High enough fluences with pulse durations equal to thermal relaxation time (TRT) will limit diffusion of heat from the target vessels and cause photocoagulation. Excessive long pulse durations, longer than the thermal relaxation time, can lead to diffusion of thermal damage to surrounding tissue. In contrast, excessively short durations can cause excessive purpura

TABLE 2: Spot diameter should be 10 times the size of lesion, to have no geometrical loss

Epidermal lesions (0.1 mm)	1 mm
Port-wine stain (1 mm)	10 mm
Tattoos (2 mm)	20 mm
Hair (3 mm)	30 mm

TABLE 3: Approximate thermal relaxation time for vessels of different diameters

Diameter (µm)	Thermal relaxation time (ms)
10	0.048
20	0.19
50	1.2
100	4.8
200	19.0
300	42.6

Box 2: Factors influencing the treatment outcome
- Vessels size
- Depth of the lesion
- Area of the body involved
- Laser spot size
- Skin type
- Fluence

without necessarily causing elimination of the vessel (Table 3). As a rule **shorter pulse, durations are better for smaller vessels, whereas longer pulse durations are better for larger vessels.**[8]

Cooling: the fourth factor is cooling, it is a must to prevent epidermal damage. It should form an integral part of laser treatment to minimize collateral damage and to reduce postoperative complications like swelling, scarring and pigmentation.[9] Thus, selective cooling of the epidermis before, during, and after treatment allows higher temperatures in the target structures without causing damage to the epidermis. Direct contact cooling, forced cold air, and cryogen spray are methods adapted for cooling.[9,10]

Factors influencing treatment outcome can be device or patient specific (Box 2). The main device specific factors are spot size and fluence. Patient specific factors are as follows:
- Diameter of vessels: vessels with a diameter of 10–100 µm have TRT of 1–10 ms, whereas blood vessels with diameter >100 µm have a higher TRT, and therefore, require longer pulse duration
- Depth of lesions: superficially located lesions (papillary dermis) are treated with standard wavelengths (577, 585 nm), but the deeper vessels need longer wavelength (up to 600 nm) for deeper penetration

- Site of lesions: lesions on face and upper trunk respond better than those in lower trunk and legs. In scar prone areas and delicate skin, reduction in 10–20% of fluence is advisable. Malformations on the first and third branches of trigeminal nerve respond better than those over the second branch
- Age of patient: as the blood vessels are smaller and more superficially located, young patients respond better than elderly
- Skin type: epidermal melanin is the main competitor for laser absorption and can damage the epidermis. Hence, darker skin types require longer pulse duration, higher fluence, and longer pulse intervals.

An optimal fluence is chosen based mainly on vessel color, vessel size, intravascular pressure, and depth of lesion. Purple and blue vessels absorb more energy than pink and red vessels, and require less fluence. Greater intravascular pressure (nose or legs) require higher fluences to achieve effective thermocoagulation.

Points to Remember

- If lesion is dark-red than the surrounding tissue, a case can be made for hemoglobin selective technology
- Ratio of absorption of the vascular target versus surrounding skin should not exceed 10:1

- Wavelength selectivity should be based on optimal ratio of vascular to pigment destruction
- Large spot size minimizes polka dot effect
- Beam profile must be flat topped
- Surface cooling is by contact sapphire window/copper plate/cryogen spray/dynamic cooling device (DCD).

❏ SPECIFIC CONDITIONS

There are various indications for vascular laser that includes both congenital and acquired conditions (Box 3).

Facial Telangiectasia[2,11,12]

The improvement of telangiectasia is achieved by direct heating of hemoglobin. The choice of lasers for smaller telangiectasia (0.1–0.6 mm) are PDL/KTP and IPL (Figure 1). For larger telangiectasia of (>1 mm), the choices are long pulse Nd:YAG and alexandrite laser. Diode 940 nmis an alternative choice.

The parameters for IPL (filter—550/560/570) are fluence of 12–45 J/cm^2; double pulse width of 2.4 ms/6.0 ms and pulse delay of 10–30 ms. One should expect epidermal desquamation, if it is to be avoided, then use longer wave length or increase delay time between double/triple pulses. Advantages of IPL are lack of purpura and adverse sequelae.

The parameters for long pulsed Nd:YAG 1,064 nm are fluence of 120–170 J/cm^2, pulse width of 5–40 ms, spot size of 3–6 mm.

The parameters for diode 940 nm are fluence of 140 J/cm^2, pulse width of 20 ms, spot size of 3 mm.

Pearls

- Always use smallest spot size and smallest of fluence
- The efficacy of millisecond laser can be improved by using plastic mask to protect the surrounding skin

---

Box 3: Indications for vascular lasers[2,3]

- Capillary malformations
  - Infantile PWS
  - Macular PWS in adults
  - Hypertrophic PWS in adults
- Hemangioma
  - Superficial hemangioma
  - Mixed type hemangioma
  - Evolving hemangioma
- Venous malformations
- Telangiectasias
  - Spider angiomata
  - Actinic telangiectasia
  - CREST syndrome
  - Essential telangiectasia
  - Hereditary hemorrhagic telangiectasia
  - Radiation dermatitis
- Rosacea
  - Facial erythema
  - Associated with rosacea
- Flushing and blushing
- Cherry angiomas
- Venous lakes
- Poikiloderma of Civatte
- Miscellaneous
  - Angiokeratomas
  - Glomus tumors
  - Pyogenic granuloma
  - Blue rubber bleb nevi
  - Warts
  - Erythematous and hypertrophic scars

PWS, port-wine stain; CREST, Calcinosis, Raynaud's phenomenon, Esophageal dysmotility, Sclerodactyly, and Telangiectasia.

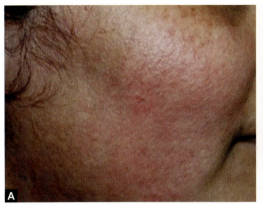
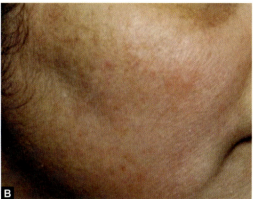

Figure 1: **A,** Facial telangiectasia; **B,** after six sessions of puled dye laser (E 6 J/cm^2, pulse width 0.45 ms, spot size 5 mm; device set parameters).

- Oxyhemoglobin absorption of 1,064 nm is 10 times lesser than 532/595, nm hence need to use high fluence
- More the spot size, greater is the scarring, hence recommended spot size is less than 2 mm.

Spider Angiomas/Telangiectasia

Laser of choice is PDL. Alternate choices are IPL with small tip adaptor and small spot KTP with parameters similar to that of facial telangiectasia.

Generalized Essential Telangiectasia

Large spot KTP is the laser of choice with fluence of 6–8 J/cm^2, spot size 10 mm, pulse width 18–22 ms, and contact cooling. Pulsed dye laser is the alternate choice with fluence of 6–7 J/cm^2 (Figure 2).[13]

Rosacea

Intense pulsed light (filter 550/560 nm) is the device of choice. The main advantage of IPL in rosacea is thermal destruction of demodex mites that contributes to the therapeutic effects of IPL. Erythema usually recurs within 6 months of laser treatment, most likely due to resurgence of demodex population and associated inflammation and hence control of disease requires maintenance treatment twice a year.[14,15] Parameters are double pulse 2.4 and 4 ms, pulse delay 10 ms, fluence 18–26 J/cm^2. The treatment interval is every 4 weeks for six to eight sessions followed by maintenance of twice a year.[15,16]

Alternate device used is PDL 595 nm. The parameters are fluence 7–9 J/cm^2, pulse width 6 ms, and cryogen spray cooling[17] (Figures 3 and 4).Resistant rosacea responds best to amino levulinic acid photodynamic therapy.[18]

Poikiloderma of Civatte[19,20]

Device of choice is IPL and alternate choices are large spot KTP, extended pulse PDL, and 1,550 nm erbium glass.

The PDL parameters are: fluence of 5–6 J/cm^2, pulse width of 1.5 ms, and spot size of 10 mm with cryospray cooling. Fluence of 7–9 J/cm^2, Pulse width of 10 to 20 ms are adapted in nonpurpuric approach (Figure 5).

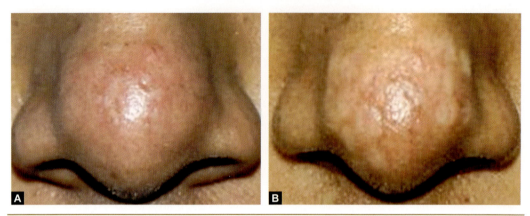

Figure 2: **A,** Generalized essential telangiectasia; **B,** after two sessions of pulsed dye laser (E 6 J/cm^2, pulse width 0.45 ms, spot size 5 mm).

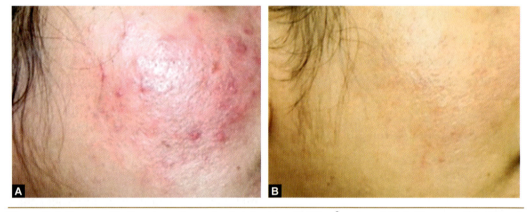

Figure 3: **A,** Rosacea; **B,** after six sessions of puled dye laser (E 5J/cm^2, pulse width 0.45 ms, spot size 5 mm).

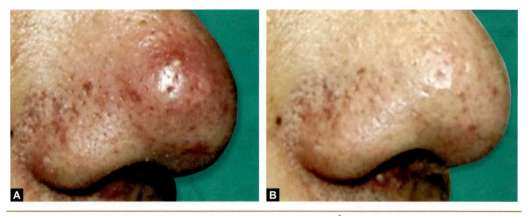

Figure 4: **A,** Rosacea; **B,** after two sessions of pulsed dye laser (E 5 J/cm^2, pulse width 0.45 ms, spot size 5 mm).

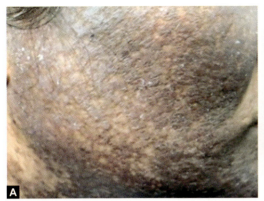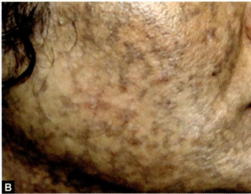

Figure 5: **A,** Poikiloderma of Civatte; **B,** after four sessions of Q-switched neodymium: yttrium-aluminum-garnet (E 4.6 J/cm^2, spot size 5 mm) + fractional carbon dioxide (E 30 mJ/cm^2, power-20 W, 100 spots/cm^2) with 11 sessions of PDL (E 5J/cm^2, pulse width 0.45 ms, spot size 5 mm) and two sessions of fractional erbium:yttrium-aluminum-garnet (E 16 J/cm^2, 2 passes, frequency 1 Hz, spot size 12 × 12 mm).

Pearls

- Demelanizing agents and hydroquinone application to detan for a month increases ratio of vascular to melanin heating leading to better efficacy and safety
- Choosing IPL has an advantage of clearing both pigment and vessels. Settings are device specific. Purpura is intravascular and resolves in 3–5 days. Footprint of contact crystal may be present for the first two sessions, patients need to be informed
- One has to keep in mind pigmentation in poikiloderma is also because of deoxyhemoglobin, because melanin and deoxyhemoglobin shares common reflectances at 560 nm, which is the deoxyhemoglobin peak.

Nevus Simplex or Salmon Patch/ Port-wine Stain

The gold standard treatment of PWS is always PDL.[9] Alternate options include new generation IPL and KTP laser. Early intervention is preferably at 3 month of birth because of smaller size of the lesion, smaller diameter of vessels, which are superficial, and also reduce permanent adverse sequelae.[21,22] Not to be used lasers are carbon dioxide, Nd:YAG, and copper vapor, but there are few indications where they can be employed.[23]

Topical anesthesia in treating PWS is better avoided as eutectic mixture of local anesthetics (EMLA) causes local vasoconstriction impeding visualization of the lesion. Prilocaine constituent of EMLA is also known to induce methemoglobinemia in children less than 6 months of age, particularly if they have hemoglobinopathies or glucose-6-phosphate dehydrogenase deficiency. General anesthesia is preferred in infants and small children.[21] One can consider angiogenesis inhibitors like topical rapamycin or propranolol which suppresses vascular endothelial growth factor and hypoxia sensitive gene-transcriptional regulators.[24,25]

The choice of PDL for pink/red PWS is 585 nm and for blue/dark red is PWS 595 nm. The parameters are fluence of 12 J/cm^2 for first pass and 10 J/cm^2 for second pass, pulse width of 1.5 ms for first pass, and 0.45 ms second pass. The pulse duration for dense PWS is 1.5 ms and for lighter PWS 0.45 ms (Figure 6).

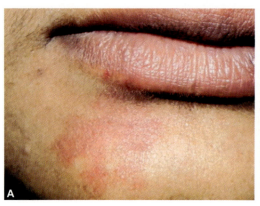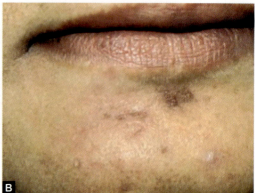

Figure 6: **A,** Port-wine stain; **B,** after eight sessions of pulsed dye laser (E 6 J/cm^2, pulse width 0.45 ms, spot size 5 mm) along with three sessions of long pulsed neodymiumdoped:yttrium-aluminum-garnet (E 140 J/cm^2, pulse width 20 ms, and spot size 3 mm).

The spot size is 7 mm with 10% overlap with cryospray/DCD. The treatment interval is 3–6 weeks for up to 8–10 sessions.[26]

The IPL parameters are first pass: fluence of 25–40 J cm^2, pulse width 10 ms, and pulse delay 60 ms. Second pass: fluence of 40–60 J/cm^2, pulse width 100 ms, pulse delay 60 ms.[9]

Aminolevulinic acid photodynamic therapy: laser used is copper vapor/CO^2 in Gaussian mode with a power of 800–1,000 W/cm^2, spot size of 9 cm and drug and light administration interval 40–55 minutes.[27,28]

Other Lasers for Resistant or Dark Port-wine Stain

Alexandrite: fluence of 25–80 J/cm^{2,} pulse width 3–20 ms, and spot size 12–15 mm. Diode: 810 nm 3.5–60 J/cm^2, spot 1 cm^2.[29,30] Neodymium: yttrium-aluminum-garnet 1,064 nm best reserved for exophytic lesions with spot size same as nodule size and fluence of 60–120 J cm^2. The endpoint is slight bluing of the lesion. Deep graying signifies over treatment and epidermal necrolyis[30,31] (Figure 7). Carbon dioxide can also be used for nodules with an advantage of coagulation of ectatic vessels.[23]

❑ GENERAL RULES IN TREATING PORT-WINE STAIN

- Treatment responses are variable due to anatomic sites, gross and microscopic anatomy of lesions and hence treatment response curve is more for lateral facial lesions > mid face lesions > nonfacial lesions
- Initial breakup of lesions allows better penetration of light in subsequent sessions
- Reasons for multiple treatments are variable depth, locational anatomy, and angiogenesis in between treatment sessions
- Multiple passes of longer pulses, progressing to shorter pulses in subsequent passes within 30 minutes interval could be the key to early clearance of lesion
- Expect atrophic scars at laser impact sites (laser imprint; Figure 8) in some cases indicating excessive delivery of energy, absence of cooling, spot overlap, and post-treatment trauma
- Side effects or blistering, crusting, scarring hypertrophic/atrophic and pigmentary changes
- Take before and after photographs
- Perform test spot of about 4–8 laser pulses
- Average number of treatment in children up to 14 years is 4–8, and in adults, it is minimum 6–20 treatments.

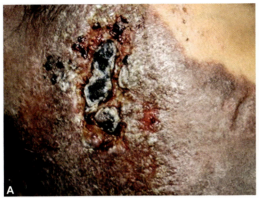
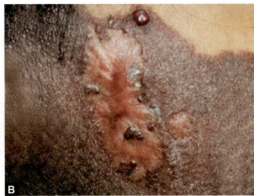

Figure 7: A, Epidermal necrolysis following long pulse neodymium:yttrium-aluminum-garnet; **B,** healing with atrophic scarring.

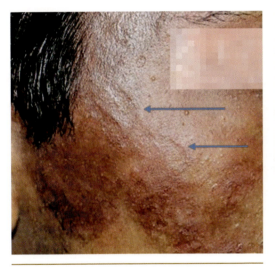

Figure 8: Laser imprint.

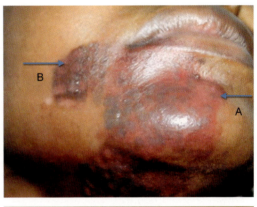

Figure 9: A, Ideal end point; **B,** ash gray color indicating over treatment.

Note

- Smaller, superficial vessels: green-yellow light
- Deeper larger vessels: longer wavelength/ long pulse duration
- Endpoint with green-yellow light is purpura (Figure 9A)
- Swelling and perceptible erythema can occur with other lasers
- Ash gray color indicates over treatment (Figure 9B).

Hemangiomas

The only indication with predicable results till today is ulcerative lesion with active ulcer PDL with 5 to 7 J/cm² with cryogen cooling minimizes further ulceration (Figures 10 and 11). Mean number of treatment sessions are two. The use of PDL for uncomplicated proliferative hemangiomas is controversial. The limitations are focal scarring, diffuse ulceration, pain, cost, and questionable impact on deep lesions.[9,32]

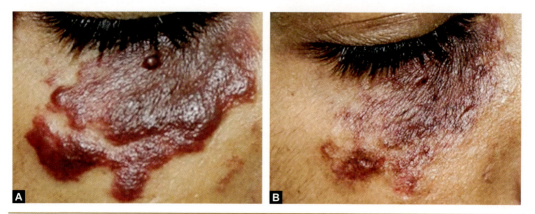

Figure 10: **A,** Hemangioma; **B,** after 15 sessions of pulsed dye laser (E 5 J/cm^2, pulse width 0.45 ms, spot size 5 mm) with 2 sessions of long pulsed neodymium:yttrium-aluminum-garnet (E 120 J/cm^2, pulse width 20 ms, spot size 3 mm).

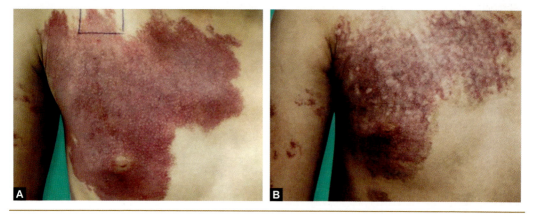

Figure 11: **A,** Hemangioma; **B,** After four sessions of pulsed dye laser (E 6 J/cm^2, pulse width 0.45 ms, spot size 5 mm).

Spider Angiomas/Telangiectasia

Laser of choice is PDL. Alternate choices are IPL with small tip adaptor and small spot KTP with parameters similar to that of facial telangiectasia. (Figure 13)

❑ MISCELLANEOUS CONDITIONS

Some miscellaneous conditions are given in Table 4.

❑ CONCLUSION

Undoubtedly vascular lasers are the treatment of choice for congenital and acquired cutaneous vascular lesions. Appropriate treatment begins with the correct diagnosis. The choice of device type and treatment parameters must be set according to the type of lesion being treated. Vessel size and depth, blood flow, skin type, melanin content, and recent suntan must be assessed prior to treatment. Available

TABLE 4: Miscellaneous indications

Indications	Laser	Spot size (mm)	Fluence (J/cm²)	Pulse width (ms)	Comments
Venous lakes[9]					Slight pressure on hand piece for better absorption and penetration of laser
Smaller lesion	KTP/PDL				
Bigger lesion	Alexandrite	6	60–80	3	
	Nd:YAG (Figure 12)	3–5	50–100	35–60	
Glomus tumor[33]	Nd:YAG	3	120–200	50	Larger the lesion smaller is the fluence and smaller the lesion larger the fluence
Blue rubber bleb nevus[9]	Nd:YAG	2–4	80–130	50	
Angiofibromas/ fibrous papules[34]	Carbon dioxide (Figure 14)	Continu-ous mode	2–5 watts (power)		
Striae rubra[9]	PDL	7–10	5–6	1.5	
Sebaceous hyperplasia[41]	PDL	3	15	1.5	Stacked pulses at 1.5 Hz. Endpoint is yellow to gray color
Ecchymosis[35]	PDL	6–10	5–6	10	
Molluscum contagiosum[36]	PDL	7	6–7	6.45	
Warts[37,38]	PDL	5–7	12–15		Give 2–4 passes without cooling to achieve the endpoint of grayish discoloration. Flat lesions require lower fluence and 1–2 passes only
	IPL		30–45	10	Use hole punch index card for better clearance and surrounding skin protection
Lymphangioma circumscriptum[39]	PDL				Blue/red lesions are amenable for PDL
Pyogenic granuloma[40]	PDL	3	6–9		The lesion is compressed with glass slide and treated.
	Nd:YAG	3–7	100–250	20–50	Carbon dioxide vaporization works best for pyogenic granuloma

Continued

Continued

TABLE 4: Miscellaneous indications					
Indications	Laser	Spot size (mm)	Fluence (J/cm^2)	Pulse width (ms)	Comments
Post-fillers bruises/ scars/vascular keloids[41] (Figures 15 and 16)	PDL	6–10	4–6	6–10	Clears within 1–3 days with IPL treatment. Parameters of minimum purpuric settings are to be employed

KTP, potassium titanyl phosphate; PDL, pulsed dye laser; Nd:YAG, neodymium:yttrium-aluminum-garnet; IPL, intense pulsed light.

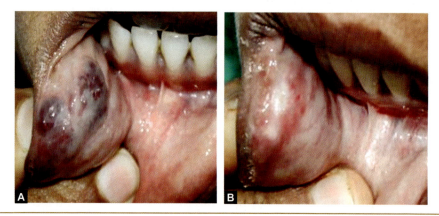

Figure 12: A, Venous lakes; **B,** after one session of long pulsed neodymiumdoped:yttrium-aluminum-garnet (E 220 J/cm^2, pulse width 40 ms, spot size 3 mm).

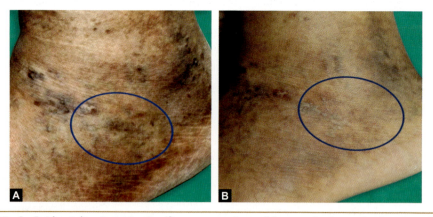

Figure 13: A, Spider telangiectasia; **B,** after one session of long pulsed neodymiumdoped:yttrium-aluminum-garnet (E 240 J/cm^2, pulse width 40 ms, spot size 3 mm).

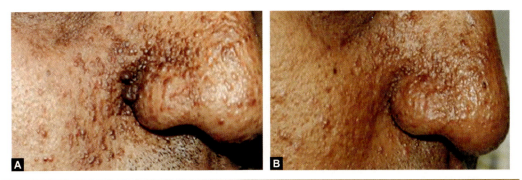

Figure 14: A, Angiofibromas; **B,** after three sessions of ablative carbon dioxide laser (E 60 mJ/cm^2, power 30 W, pulse rate 40 Hz) along with two sessions of microablative erbium:yttrium-aluminum-garnet (E 10–15 J/cm^2, spot size 2 mm).

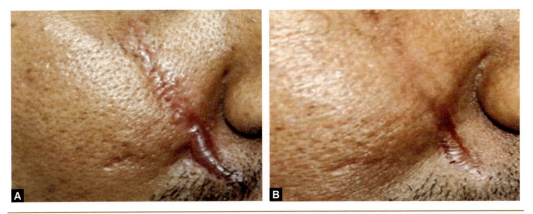

Figure 15: A, Hypertrophic scar; **B,** after four sessions of PDL (E 5 J/cm^2, pulse width-0.45 ms, spot size 5 mm).

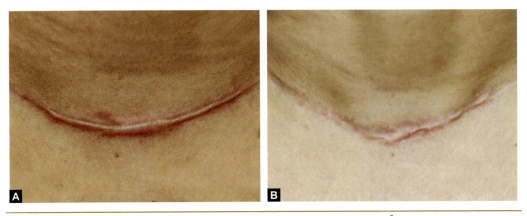

Figure 16: A, Vascular keloid; **B,** after five sessions of pulsed dye laser (E 4 J/cm^2, pulse width 0.45 ms, spot size 5 mm).

vascular lasers are more suitable for Western skin types and the parameters used in Western skin may not always suit all other skin types. The technology keeps rapidly evolving and hence guidelines are reviewed periodically. We present the current guidelines and parameters for various disorders and devices while sharing our experience in using vascular lasers on Indian skin.

❑ REFERENCES

1. Anderson RR, Parrish JA. Microvasculature can be selectively damaged using dye lasers: a basic theory and experimental evidence in human skin. Lasers Surg Med. 1981;1:263-76.

2. Ross EV, Krakowski AC. Laser treatment for vascular laser. In: Mitchel P. Goldman, Richard Fitzpatrick, Victor Ross and Suzanne L. Kilmer. Lasers and energy devices for the skin. 2nd ed. CRP Press; 2013.

3. Kauvar An, Troilius A, Robinson JK. Laser and light treatment of acquired and congenital vascular lesions. Text book of Surgery of Skin. 2nd edition. 563-79.

4. Dai T, Pikkula BM, Wang LV, Anvari B. Comparison of human skin opto-thermal response to near-infrared and visible laser irradiations: a theoretical investigation. Phys Med Biol. 2004;49(21):4861-77.

5. Basschaart N, Faber DJ, van Leeuwen TG, Alders MC. In vivo low coherence spectroscopic measurements of local hemoglobin in absorption spectra in human skin. J Biomed Opt. 2011:16:100-504.

6. Keijzer M, Pickering JW, van Gemert MJ. Laser beam diameter for port wines stain treatment. Laser Surg Med. 1991:11:601-5.

7. Lucassen GW, Verkruysse W, Keijzer M, van Gemert MJ. Light distributions in port-wine stain model containing multiple cylindrical and curved blood vessels. Lasers Surg Med. 1996;18:345-57.

8. Kimel S, Svaasand LO, Cao D, Hammer-Wilson MJ, Nelson JS. Vascular response to laser photothermolysis as a function of pulse duration, vessel type, and diameter: Implications for port wine stain laser therapy. Lasers Surg Med. 2002;30(2):160-9.

9. Nelson JS, Milner TE, Anvari B, Tanenbaum BS, Svaasand LO, Kimel S. Dynamic epidermal cooling in conjunction with laser induced photothermolysis of port wine stain blood vessels. Lasers Surg Med. 1996;19:224.

10. Anvari B, Milner TE, Tanenbaum BS, Kimel S, Svaasand LO, Nelson JS. Selective cooling of biological tissues: application for thermally medicated therapeutic procedures. Phys Med Biol. 1995;40:241-52.

11. Goldberg DJ, Marcus J. The use of the frequency-doubled Q switched Nd:YAG laser in the treatment of small cutaneous vascular lesions. Dermatol Surg. 1996;22: 841-4.

12. Kauvar AN, Rosen N, Khrom T. A newly modified 595-nm pulsed dye laser with compression hand piece for the treatment of photo damaged skin. Laser Surg Med. 2006;38:808-13.

13. Goldman MP, Bennett RG. Treatment of telangiectasia: a review. J Am Acad Dermatol. 1987;17(2 Pt 1):167-82.

14. Schmidt N, Gans E. Demodex and rosacea I: the prevalence and numbers of Demodex mites in rosacea. Cosmetic Dermatol. 2004;17:497-502.

15. Schroeter CA, Haaf-von Below S, Neumann HA. Effective treatment of rosacea using intense pulsed light systems. Dermatol Surg. 2005;31:1285-9.

16. Menezes N, Moreira A, Mota G, Bapista A. Quality of life and rosacea: pulse dye laser impact. J Cosmet Laser Ther. 2009;11:139-41.

17. Jasim ZF, Woo WK, Handley JM. Long-pulsed (6-ms) pulsed dye laser treatment of rosacea-associated telangiectasia using subpurpuric clinical threshold. Dermatol Surg. 2004;30:37-40.

18. Baglieri F, Scuderi G. Treatment of recalcitrant granulomatous rosacea with ALA-PDT: report of case. Indian J Dermatol Venereol Leprol. 2011;77;356.

19. Weiss RA, Goldman MP, Weiss MA. Treatment of poikiloderma of Civatte with an intense pulsed light source. Dermatol Surg. 2000;26:823-7; discussion 828.

20. Goldman MP, Weiss RA. Treatment of poikiloderma of Civatte on the neck with an intense pulsed light source. Plast Reconstr Surg. 2001;107:1376-81.

21. Stier MF, Click SA, Hirsch RJ. Laser treatment of pediatric vascular lesions: port wine stains and hemangiomas. J Am Acad Dermatol. 2008;58:261-85.

22. Chapas AM, Eickhorst K, Geronemus RG. Effective of early treatment of facial port wine stains in newborns: a review of 49 cases. Laser Surg Med. 2007;39:563-5.

23. Buecker JW, Ratz JL, Richfield DF. Histology of port-wine stains treated with carbon dioxide laser. J Am Acad Dermatol. 1984;10:1014-9.

24. Jia W, Sun V, Tran N, Choi B, Liu SW, Mihm MC Jr, et al. Long term blood vessel removal with combined laser and topical rapamycin anti angiogenic therapy: implication for effective port wine stain treatment. Laser Surg Med. 2010;42:105-12.

25. Moehrle M, Leaute-Labreze C, Schmidt V, Röcken M, Poets CF, Goelz R. Topical timolol for small hemangiomas of infancy. Pediatr Dermatol. 2013;30(2):245-9.

26. Goldman MP, Fitzpatrick RE, Ruiz-Esparza J. Treatment of port-wine stains (capillary malformation) with the flash lamp-pumped pulsed dye laser. J Pediatr. 1993;122:71-7.

27. Lu YG, Wu JJ, Yang YD, Yang HZ, He Y. Photodynamic therapy of port wine stains. J Dermatolog Treat. 2010;21:240-4.

28. Huang N, Cheng G Li X, Gu Y, Liu F, Zhong Q, et al. Influence of drug-light interval on photodynamic therapy of port wine stains simulation and validation of mathematic models. Photodiagnosis Photodynther. 2008;5;120-6.

29. Jasim ZF, Handley JM. Treatment of pulsed dye laser-resistant port wine stain birthmarks. J Am Acad Dermatol. 2007;57:677-82.

30. Izikson L, Nelson JS, Anderson RR. Treatment of hypertrophic and resistant port wine stain with a 755 nm laser: a case series of 20 patients. Laser Surg Med. 2009;41:427-32.

31. Geronemus RG. Long pulsed neodymium:yttrium-aluminum-garnet laser treatment for port wine stains. J Am Acad Dermatol. 2006;54:923.

32. Morelli JG, Tan OT, Weston WL. Treatment of uncreated hemangiomas with the pulsed tunable dye lasers. Am J Dis Child. 1991;145:1062-4.

33. Hughes R, Lacour JP, Chiaverini C, Rogopoulos A, Passerson T. Nd-YAG Laser treatment for multiple cutaneous glomangiomas: report of 3 cases. Arch Dermatol. 2011;147:255-6.

34. Weiss ET, Geronemus RG. New technique using combined pulsed dye laser and fractional resurfacing for treating facial angiofibromas in tuberous sclerosis. Laser Surg Med. 2010;42;357-60.

35. Karen JK, Hale EK, Geronemus RG. A simple solution to the common problem of ecchymosis. Arch Dermatol. 2010;146:94-5.

36. Binder B, Weger W, Kemericki P, Kopera D. Treatment of molluscum contagiosum with pulsed dye laser: pilot study with 19 children. Dermatol Surg. 2008;6:121-5.

37. Sethuraman G, Richards KA, Herimagalore RN, Wagner A. Effectiveness of pulsed dye laser in treatment of recalcitrant warts in children. Dermatol Surg. 2010;36:58-65.

38. Tan OT, Hurwitz RM, Stafford TJ. Pulsed dye laser treatment of recalcitrant verrucae: a preliminary report. Lasers Surg Med. 1993;13:127-37.

39. Lai CH, Hanson SG, Mallory SB. Lymphangioma circumscriptum treated with pulsed dye laser. Pediatr Dermatol. 2001;18:509-10.

40. Gonzalez S, Vibhagool C, Falo LD Jr, Momtaz KT, Grevelink J, González E. Treatment of pyogenic granulomas with the 585-nm pulsed dye laser. J Am Acad Dermatol. 1996;35:428-31.

41. Goldman MP, editor. Lasers and energy devices for the skin. 2nd ed.; 2013.

Complications of Laser Hair Reduction

K Narendra Kamath, Hema Mallya, Vindhya A Pai

❑ INTRODUCTION

It is an increasing concern among women and men to remove excess unwanted hair. In women, the increase in hair growth on most androgen sensitive sites (e.g., upper lip, chin, mid sternum, upper abdomen, back, and buttocks) is known as hirsutism. It affects 5–10% of women of reproductive age, and most women have associated polycystic ovarian syndrome (PCOS).

❑ EVALUATION OF WOMEN WITH HIRSUTISM[1]

Hair growth can be graded as either normal or excessive based upon the Ferriman-Gallwey score. Using this method, nice androgen sensitive sites are graded from 0 to 4.

There are limitations to this grading as the expression of hair growth varies between racial/ethnic groups. Most East Asian women have little body hair, White and Afro-American women have an intermediate amount, and most Mediterranean, South Asian, and Middle Eastern women have substantially higher quantities of body hair, in spite of serum androgen concentrations being similar in all groups showing a modest correlation between the hair growth and serum androgen.[2] This shows the role of androgen levels apart, local factors and end-organ sensitivity to circulating androgens also is variable.[3]

❑ CAUSES OF INCREASED HAIR GROWTH AND INDICATIONS FOR LASER HAIR REDUCTION[2]

- Lanugo hair: androgen independent, lightly pigmented vellus hair seen on the face
- Hypertrichosis: the excessive growth of androgen-independent hair (i.e. vellus), prominent in nonsexual areas and most commonly familial or caused by systemic disorders like hypothyroidism, anorexia nervosa, malnutrition, porphyria, dermatomyositis, or medications (phenytoin, penicillamine, diazoxide, minoxidil, cyclosporine)
- Hirsutism—causes include:
  ○ Polycystic ovarian disease (Figure 1)
  ○ Idiopathic hirsutism
  ○ Congenital adrenal hyperplasia
  ○ Ovarian tumors
  ○ Adrenal tumors
  ○ Cushing's disease

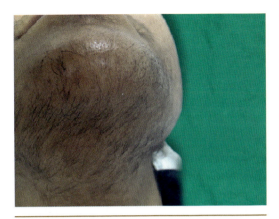

Figure 1: Hirsutism in a patient with polycystic ovarian disease.

- ○ Hyperthecosis
- ○ Drugs like danazol (commonly used in the past for endometriosis)
- ○ Hyperinsulinemia and insulin resistance[3,4]
- • Others: pilonidal sinus, recurrent folliculitis in flexures, pseudofolliculitis, ingrown hair.

Male Patients

This newer subgroup has demands for removal of ear hair (more in South India), nasal surface hair, surplus hair on malar area, truncal and chest hair, beard shaping, frontal shaping of bald scalp/after hair transplantation, finger hair, body hair in body builders/models, metrosexuals.

Transgender

Removal of masculine hair patterns for complete feminization.

Mentally Challenged

Removal of body hair especially pubic and axillary (as an extended measure in body hygiene maintenance) on the basis of consent by family members is a debatable issue. A legal advice is best taken before venturing in this territory.

❑ EQUIPMENT AVAILABLE

The procedure is done with any of the devices given in table 1.

Pain Free Lasers[6]

- • Pneumatic skin flattening: it works by coupling a vacuum chamber to generate negative pressure and to flatten the skin against the hand piece treatment window. Based on the gate theory of pain transmission, it stimulates pressure receptors in the skin immediately prior to firing of the laser pulse, thereby blocking activation of pain fibers. Faster, painless treatment may be achieved.
- • IN-motion technology: a unique IN-motion technology which combines concurrent cooling with a gradual thermal rise to the

TABLE 1: Commonly used devices for laser hair reduction			
Device wavelength	Skin types	Advantages	Disadvantages
1064 nm Nd:YAG	1–4	Good for darker skin types	Pain, possible folliculitis
755 nm alexandrite	1–3	Good for lighter hair	Pain, possible folliculitis
810 nm diode	1–5	Good for darker skin	Pain, possible folliculitis
IPL	1-5	Less expensive	Not as effective as laser systems, paradoxical hair stimulation[5]

Nd:YAG, neodymium-doped yttrium aluminum garnet; IPL, intense pulsed light.

target's therapeutic temperature without the risk of injury, and with much less pain for the patient. This is in contrast to the high peak energies used in traditional diode lasers that requires high cooling before, during and after each pulse and requires that the hand piece remains stationary during energy delivery. The sweeping technique of IN-motion technology enables continuous management of a larger treatment area for increased comfort and fewer missed spots.

Contraindications

- Patients with suntan: best counseled about the risk of worsening of hyperpigmentation over procedural areas, and hence the procedure may be deferred by at least 2 weeks
- Patients with unrealistic expectation: they are best discouraged about the procedure even if not convinced after comprehensive counseling. These patients may be a deterrent to the surgeon's skills, and can be bad brand ambassadors
- Patients on isotretinoin
- Patients having history of herpes infection type 1: active lesions presence is a definite contraindication, while suspect history or naïve patients are best given a course of prophylactic acyclovir after counselling. If not, a patient may attribute the primary and recurrent attacks to the procedure
- Patients having predominantly white hair: melanin is the chromophore, and its absence in gray hair makes them refractory to lasers. Alternate methods may be planned for these later
- Patients with photosensitive disorders
- Pregnancy and lactation: lasers being newer entities, and lack of long-term studies limit its usage
- Mentally challenged patients: this group has been discussed earlier

- Retroviral disease: microtrauma during preparation calls for caution and restraint
- Age group: requests arise from parents to have the procedure on their preteen children. Experience in this age group is limited all over.

❑ STEPS TO BE TAKEN BEFORE THE HAIR REMOVAL LASER IS DONE

- Ask for menstrual history in females—regular or irregular. If irregular then look for the signs of PCOS. Polycystic ovarian syndrome is a common endocrine disorder among women who are of reproductive age group. The cutaneous features of PCOS are hirsutism, acanthosis nigricans, acne, and alopecia. In patients with PCOS, there will be high levels of luteinizing hormone (LH), testosterone, and low levels of follicle-stimulating hormone (FSH) in the blood
- Do a blood check up on the 5th day of the menstrual cycle to detect the levels of LH, FSH, and testosterone. Patients with PCOS will have LH/FSH >2:1.

Procedure

- Calibrations vary amongst technologies and companies as well. The user is hence advised to familiarize oneself with the same. A short course on machine operations may be requested before purchase, and also a week long hands-on training at a reputed center
- A stand-alone laser hair removal machine is good for an established dermatologist or one totally in aesthetic practice. These machines are expensive though. A novice may buy a platform device, as it serves many other functions too
- Patient selection is of utmost importance in achieving a comprehensive success. Patients often correlate the laser hair removal to a beauty parlor procedure.

The following points are to be borne in mind by every laser surgeon:

- Counseling: good, adequate approach means a convince patient, and that always spells success
- Patient should understand that it is a "hair reduction", not "hair removal" procedure
- Rejection rates may vary from 10–30%. Do not take up every patient that requests for the procedure. Be aware of complications and litigations
- Personalize: operate by yourself if possible; if not, have a qualified doctor assistant. Usage of para staff converts to a higher quantum of failures. Plan your operation theater time, and do procedures by prior appointments. Do not mix up with general appointments, as one may lose future clients who have come just to meet the surgeon
- Ensure that the patient follows the appointment schedules correctly. Leisurely casual approach always leads to poor results
- Evaluate every female patient for hormonal dyscrasia. Hormonal aberrations calls for a multispecialty approach, and the help of a gynecologist or physician/endocrinologist is essential. In hormonal disturbances, it is better to defer the procedure by a couple of months as the hormones may delay/impede with response to lasers[4]
- In diode and alexandrite laser usage, explain about the need for preprocedure shaving. In patients who have waxed or plucked hairs recently, it is advisable to wait for a week as these procedures cause varied damage to hair bulb apparatus. An intact hair bulb always means good quantum of the chromophore. In people with a stubble, it is advisable to shave just prior to the procedure.
- Preprocedure consent is best taken every time, though the techniques are noninvasive. Preprocedure pictures are taken for documentation. Publishing the same may need prior permission. Follow privacy laws during photography and later usage of pictures.
- Laser operation theater should be dust and pest free. Lighting source should be adequate, and a light music in the background is always relaxing. Emergency fire dousing measures are to be kept handy
- Emergency kits are best available to manage any unforeseen complications. Newer guidelines advise having a functional defibrillator in the operation theater
- Super hair removal by diode needs cooled jelly to act as a cooling medium, and faster procedural execution[6] (Figure 2). Mark the areas to be operated upon by using a colored lip liner pencil (Figure 3). Shaved area with jelly on surface will surely deter the procedure with erythema setting in some patients. The color markings may be erased by usage of available specific cleansers. Never use a black/dark colored pencil, as these colors may act as chromophores and cause surface burns (Figure 4)
- Any hair tips or broken hairs on surface of operating area may absorb energy and

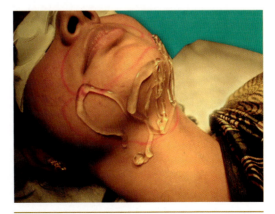

Figure 2: Ultrasound jelly application in operational area.

cause a burning smell. These hair bits are best cleared with the sticky surface of a micropore plaster.

Procedure is best initiated after adequate preparations. Laser surgeon and assistant are advised to wear the provided protective eye wear, which often is laser specific. Lacrimation

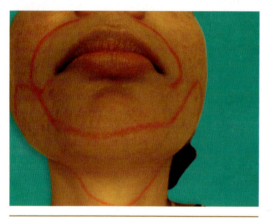

Figure 3: Skin area marked for procedure.

is an unwanted complication. Patient is made to wear the necessary provided external eye shield. Eyebrow procedures need an eye surface shield to prevent uncomfortable eye flashes.

Laser shots are best tailor-made for every patient, and every laser surgeon learns the same by experience. Many newer machines have simpler calibrations, and one needs to set the dose of laser (Joules), and final total dose (kilojoules). Machines set by self for number of seconds after one has selected the mode of delivery in continuous pattern or a variable stack pattern (2–5 stacks). Continuous mode is good on trunk, chest, limbs, while lower stacks are for sensitive areas of body. Higher stacks are helpful on face and neck. It is advisable to use stack mode in dark skinned patients.

On adequate procedure, one may observe the hair roots puffing as a result of laser energy being absorbed by melanin, and this raises the hair root temperatures to have detrimental

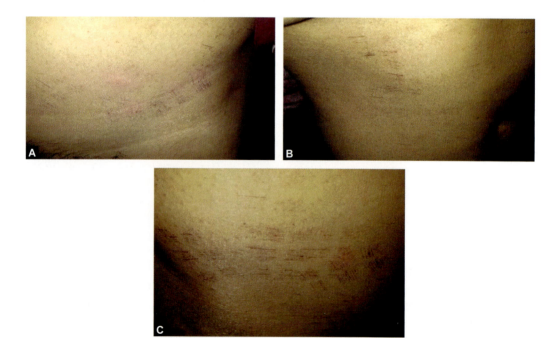

Figure 4: Superficial burns in a patient after using vacuum assisted device

effects and destruction of root. The effect every time is just on 15–20% of existing hairs. On over doing of the procedure, laser energy dissipating into vicinity causes a gentle hot feeling in some patients. One may avoid the area to prevent any burns. Recruitment of laser favorable hairs needs a month, and over multiple sittings one observes a 93–97% of reduction. Procedure is best done on a monthly basis for 6–8 sittings totally. Patients with PCOS and darker skin may need a couple extra sittings.

Five to seven days after procedure patients may complain about good hair growth at site of procedure. This actually is the extrusion of lased hair with root. Gently rubbing with a bath towel causes dropping of dark dots.

It is advisable to call patients every 3 months for a review and "touch up" as there may be a vellus hair recruitment to terminal hair. Doubtful PCOS patients are best screened afresh.

Patients are advised to avoid intense sunlight exposure for a fortnight later. Some surgeons adopt usage of lasers and waxing alternately on a fortnightly basis. This has shown satisfactory response in thick haired patients.

Technical Difficulties

- Noncompliant patients are best handled tactfully, and discouraged from future procedures
- Ingrown hairs are first needled out, and then prepared for the procedure
- Gray haired individuals are best informed of the effect only on black hairs, and are discouraged if number of gray hairs are more (Figure 5). Melatonin preparations are advised by some groups to darken the gray hairs for months as a preparatory measure. No documented reports were found

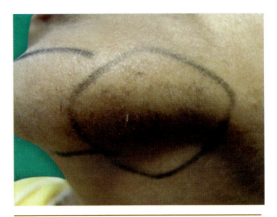

Figure 5: Persistence of gray hair.

- Nasal orifice: Presence of intranasal hairs provides challenges while operating in the philtrum region. Nasal orifice is loosely packed with cotton, to prevent laser heating the nasal hairs and causing extreme discomfort
- Introitus: Natural occurrence of more pigmentation does cause severe pain and intolerance. It is better to apply multilayers of micropore plaster slivers on the introital opening, and operate at lower doses in lower stacks.

❑ COMPLICATIONS AND MANAGEMENT

- Common skin responses are pain and discomfort. These can be minimized with appropriate dosing. Darker patients are most susceptible to this complication. Avoidance of sunlight, cold washes, and analgesics should suffice. Steroids creams may be used later. Severe burns need to be managed as a first degree burn
- Folliculitis may occur as a result of shaving, bacterial invasion, or perifollicular inflammation as a local response to laser damage (Figure 6)

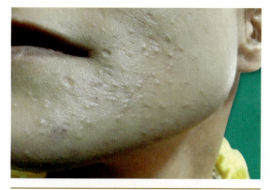

Figure 6: Folliculitis in a patient after using diode laser.

cause the same, and is often embarrassing. A wooden candy stick is gently pushed into the fornix to even out the skin at the area, and laser is done. This clears the hairs adequately (Figure 8)

- Pigmentary disturbances: Perifollicular pigmentation is common because of a probable implosion of hair roots after chromophore heat up. Perilabial pigmentation may occur if one trudges upon the vermilion border of the lips (Figures 9 and 10). Pigmentary changes are self-limiting

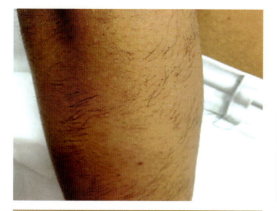

Figure 7: After six sittings with vacuum assisted diode laser—patchy coarse hair growth still present.

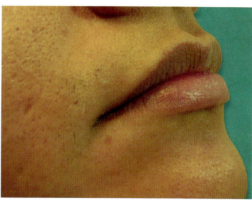

Figure 8: Chinese moustache appearance at angle of mouth.

- Paradoxical hair stimulation:[5] this complication commonly occurs in treatment with intense pulsed light due to inadequate cooling, and the heat can lead to increased hair growth (Figure 7). Patient selection is very important. Lasing on patients with vellus hairs increases the incidence. Hair may turn to terminal, increasing length of vellus hair, increased appearance are common in indiscreetly done procedures
- Chinese moustache appearance: It is the persistence of hairs near the angle of the mouth. Natural topographic variations

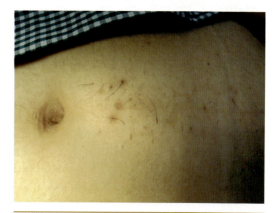

Figure 9: Perifollicular pigmentation in absence of infection.

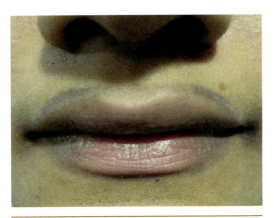

Figure 10: Pigmentation of vermilion border of lips.

- Pigmented nevi: avoid operating upon the same, and do not attempt hair removal from a hairy nevus. Intractable pain, and unforeseen complications may be seen.

❑ CONCLUSION

Cases having severe hirsutism or hirutism with associated acne often pose therapeutic challenges. It is always advisable to rule out PCOS or ovarian tumor (in relevant cases) before starting any laser procedure (Figures 11 and 12).

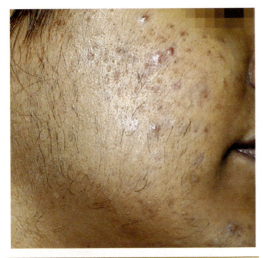

Figure 11: Moderate acne with hirsutism indicates underlying polycystic ovarian syndrome.

Courtesy: Derma-Care, Mangaluru

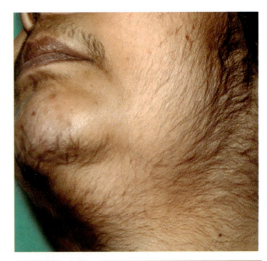

Figure 12: Severe hirsutism: ovarian tumor must be ruled out.

Courtesy: Derma-Care, Mangaluru

❑ REFERENCES

1. Ferriman D, Gallwey JD. Clinical assessment of body hair growth in women. J Clin Endocrinol Metab. 1961;21: 1440-7.
2. Lipton MG, Sherr L, Elford J, Rustin MH, Clayton WJ. Women living with facial hair: the psychological and behavioral burden. J Psychosom Res. 2006;61:161-8.
3. Carmina E, Koyama T, Chang L, Stanczyk FZ, Lobo RA. Does ethnicity influence the prevalence of adrenal hyperandrogenism and insulin resistance in polycystic ovary syndrome? Am J Obstet Gynecol. 1992;167: 1807-12.
4. Kirschner MA, Samojlik E, Silber D. A comparison of androgen production and clearance in hirsute and obese women. J Steroid Biochem. 1983;19:607-14.
5. Alajlan A, Shapiro J, Rivers JK, MacDonald N, Wiggin J, Lui H. Paradoxical hypertrichosis after laser epilation. J Am Acad Dermatol. 2005;53:85-8.
6. Olsen EA. Methods of hair removal. J Am Acad Dermatol. 1999;40:143-55.

Complications in Intense Pulsed Light Treatment

Avitus JR Prasad

❑ INTRODUCTION

Intense pulsed light (IPL) devices are nonlaser high intensity light sources that produces a broad wavelength output of noncoherent light, usually in the 400–1,200 nm range when burst of electric current passes through a high intensity xenon gas-filled flash lamp.[1] The lamp output is then directed toward the distal end of the handpiece, which, in turn, releases the energy pulse onto the surface of the skin via a sapphire or quartz crystal block. Individual systems use different cooling systems, such as a cryogen spray, contact cooling, or forced refrigerated air, to protect the epidermis in contact with the conduction crystal of the handpiece.[2]

The first IPL device obtained Food and Drug Administration clearance in 1995 for treatment of lower extremity telangiectasias. Since then, its favorable cost and versatility in contrast to many single-spectrum lasers, has led to its rapid proliferation and use in a number of different clinical settings. Despite early claims of having too many side effects and too little efficacy, innovations in technology have resulted in the development of more powerful, predictable, and reliable devices enhancing their usefulness in skin rejuvenation.

In contrast to most lasers, the light pulse duration of IPL systems can easily be changed to match the thermal relaxation time of the target. Most lasers emit a single, characteristic wavelength, whereas flash lamps in IPL systems emit the entire visual optical spectrum as well as a part of the near infrared spectrum from 400–1,200 nm.

A band of wavelengths matching the target's absorption spectrum can readily be obtained by selecting an appropriate combination of optical filters. Intense pulsed light systems have been shown to be clinically equal and in some cases superior to laser systems (for pulse durations >2.5 ms) when the primary mode of action is photothermolysis.

This chapter gives an overview of the strategies needed to avoid complications in IPL treatment. Intense pulsed light, like most lasers, have its share of complications. Most of the complications can be prevented, some need salvage, and some should have been avoided by not performing the procedure in the first place.

Unfortunately, IPL equipment increasingly are being used with no supervision by persons with no medical qualifications, and in some cases the doctor do not have the complete knowledge about the working mechanisms and technical know how about the machines. Many doctors buy it for the reason that it is a cheaper solution and that some of his colleagues or peers are having the technology. Intense pulsed light treatments are performed without training and proper understanding about its parameters.

❑ FACTORS TO BE CONSIDERED AS A PREREQUISITE FOR THE DOCTOR OR AESTHETIC ASSISTANT

Training

Inadequate training and lack of experience on the part of the doctor are the main reasons in any treatment error. In recent years, there have been many reports of laser treatments administered by personnel with no medical qualifications at all.[3]

The specialist should have good knowledge about the basics and applications of IPL to limit the incidence of complications. Proper training and hands on workshops under the guidance of peers who are experienced in IPL is very essential for a doctor who is starting to do IPL.

Only once the doctor is confident, should IPL be performed. The procedure should be done either by the specialist doctor personally or at least under his or her supervision. Training of the doctor's assistants in aiding the doctor while performing an IPL is also important.

Diagnosis

A correct diagnosis is crucial before taking up the case for IPL. A good clinical acumen can identify whether the dermatological condition will benefit from IPL. A detailed preoperative consultation, thorough examination, and stringent patient selection is needed before a planned intervention, and it ensures the use of the laser/IPL best suited to the dermatological condition.

It also includes discussing with the patient about the condition, possible therapeutic options, why one chose this option, the level of clearance which can be expected, and period of treatment. This helps in making the patient adhere to the treatment protocol and helps in building a good patient doctor relationship, which is very essential in case any untoward complications occur.

Proper medical history is needed, as for any laser treatment patient with history of currently on or having taken isotretinoin in the past 6 months, patients with unrealistic expectations should be avoided.

Knowing How to Treat Complications

Complications which could arise from various IPL treatments and conditions should be well understood. All measures should be taken in preventing complications. The doctor should be trained in identifying and treating the complications early which would in turn result in a good clinical outcome.

❑ FACTORS ABOUT THE INTENSE PULSED LIGHT WHICH SHOULD BE UNDERSTOOD TO PREVENT COMPLICATIONS

Parameters

Energy/Fluence

Theory of selective photothermolysis by Rox Anderson and Parrish[4] and the extended theory of photothermolysis by Rox Anderson and Altshuler[5] forms the basis on which IPL and lasers work. The energy chosen should be target specific, it also depends on the filter used and skin type of the patient.

Deeper chromophore will require higher fluence and higher filter. There should be upper and lower value for energy in each condition. Choosing the proper energy/fluence prevents complications. Lower fluence for darker skin and higher fluence for lighter skin. For example, if the hair removal with 690 nm filter allows fluence/energy from 28 J/cm^2 to 35 J/cm^2, start with 28 J/cm^2 for skin type V and VI and 35 J/cm^2 for skin type I and II.

Do test fires before determining the comfortable energy for the patients, always test patch with the lowest joules for that particular filter and increase by 1 J in next shots and determine the comfortable energy. For example, hair removal start with 25 J if 640 nm filter is used or 28 J if 690 nm filter is used depending on skin type. Some patients say that with 28 J they feel the heat, in some they feel heat at 34 J.

Intense pulsed light machines from different manufacturers have different energy delivery, the energy settings of one company will not be the same in another machine. Because of this nonstandard emission, one has to test fire the machine and find out the comfortable energy in a particular skin type.

Pulse Duration and Pulse Delay (On and Off Time)

Pulse duration and delay depends on thermal relaxation time[4] of the intended target and also the time required for the epidermis to cool in between the pulses to prevent epidermal burns. Pulse duration depends on different chromophores, size of the target, and depth of the target. Longer pulse durations can cause more collateral damage to tissue surrounding the intended target. Lesser pulse

delay results in epidermal injury. Ideally, 10–20 ms between pulses is required to prevent this complication.

Cooling

Cooling the skin before, during, and soon after the treatment effectively dissipates heat and allows to use higher fluences delivered at a higher repetition rate, at the same time prevent unwanted side effects and maintain the comfort of the patient.

An IPL machine having inbuilt cooling is critical to minimizing any undue pain, redness, burns, and postprocedure hyperpigmentation.

Other methods of cooling (e.g., cold air or cold gel, and ice pack) have to be used in combination with integrated cooling. Hence, any system that does not come with integrated cooling greatly increases the frequency and severity of adverse reactions.

It should be noted that there are procedures where cooling can be a cause of negative results. For example, when doing superficial vascular work such as rosacea, postacne redness, and fine telangiectasias, precooling more than 1–2 seconds causes the superficial blood vessels to constrict and reduces the available chromophore, the oxy-, and deoxyhemoglobin which is very much needed for the success of any vascular work, thereby affecting the end result of the treatment. Cooling for lentigines, epidermal melasma, etc. will affect the outcome as the target has to be heated for results and cooling creates a problem.

The appropriate use of cooling with understanding of how much contact cooling time depending on the condition being treated is required for a successful treatment without side effects.

When cooling is applied, it should be the same amount of time in between shots. For example, in hair removal, if contact cooling is for 4 seconds and the joules used is comfortable for the patient and if the operator in the subsequent shots cools for 3 seconds in a hurry to finish the procedure, it might lead to burns.

Filters

The choice of filter depends on the target chromophore and the depth at which the chromophore is present. For example, 510–530 nm filter which is in the green wavelength works on the epidermal melanin, 640–755 nm filter which is in the red wavelength is used to target the dermal melanin in the hair.

To activate a particular wavelength, sufficient energy has to be used. A 530 nm green light will reach optimum therapeutic efficacy to target the melanin chromophore in the epidermis and upper dermis only when energy of 15–25 J/cm^2 is used depending on skin type and the IPL machine. When a 690 nm red light is used to target the mid-dermis melanin in the hair, an energy of 25–35 J/cm^2 is needed. Higher the filter used, higher the energy required to activate it.

Radiofrequency Incorporated Intense Pulsed Light

In recent years, the use of IPL with radiofrequency (RF) has become the next generation IPL treatment. This technology incorporates RF energy with IPL. The rationale behind a combination system such is that there is a synergistic interaction between the two forms of energy. The optical component selectively preheats the target through selective photothermolysis, and the RF energy is driven to the target site by the electrical conductivity of the target tissue as well as the increased conductivity generated from the optical preheating.

Intense pulse laser action on the target tissue creates an initial relatively small temperature gradient, and by applying RF energy next, a larger temperature gradient is obtained. This allows heating of the target to a sufficiently high temperature to destroy the target without heating the surrounding skin tissues to damaging levels.

A synergistic effect is obtained when the light energy component is used to heat the target tissue, which is followed by the RF component to selectively heat the desired target. This synergy allows lower levels of both types of energy to be used, thus minimizing adverse effects.

It should be noted that the RF used is nonablative and not the ablative mode.

❑ COMPLICATIONS

There are two types of complications, namely, immediate postoperative complications and delayed complications (Table 1).

Immediate Postoperative Complications

Burns

Post-IPL burns is one of the commonest complications encountered. This complications can be identified within 5 minutes of doing the procedure.

Reasons for this complications are listed below.

- Operator related:
  - Wrong filter

TABLE 1: Complications	
Immediate postoperative complications	**Delayed complications**
• Burns • Blister/vesicles formation • Erosion	• Postinflammatory hyperpigmentation • Hypopigmentation • Potential infections • Scars and keloids • Paradoxical hair growth following hair removal

- ○ Excess joules for the filter and condition
- ○ Noncontact of the crystal with the skin while firing
- ○ Sufficient cooling as per the condition and filter used was not given
- ○ Less amount of contact gel used
- ○ Failure to compensate for the energy delivered by a new machine or recently changed lamp.
- Patient related:
  - ○ Exposure to excess sunlight in the last 3–4 days prior to the procedure
  - ○ Use of cosmetics which could act as a target (chromophore) which absorb the light leading to unwanted burns
  - ○ Use of hair dye
  - ○ Patient was not honest about the comfortable joules when the test fire was done. When IPL is been performed, many patients think that if they can bear the heat produced they will get better results.

Once a burn is noticed, immediately apply ice pack or chilled saline for 10–15 minute, daily twice application of hydrocortisone or desonide mixed with fusidic acid will help in the wound healing, use of anti-inflammatory and course of azithromycin is needed.

The authors use an epidermal growth factor for the next three days to hasten wound healing and prevent delayed complications.

Blister/Vesicle Formation/Erosion

This complications follows burns in some cases mainly because of the reasons mentioned in the operator related causes.

The main reason is when the operator forgets to put in the filter before firing. Excessive joules and inadequate cooling are the other two most common reasons.

This complication is one of the hardest conditions to recover, it would take at least a period of 6–8 weeks to recover.

The sequence of healing is as follows:

- Immediate pain and burning sensation which would take 1 hour to reduce. Use of cooling pack or chilled saline is needed
- Darkening of the skin and swelling which persists for 24 hours
- Blistering and vesicles seen after 24 hours which would take 3–4 days to settle
- Erosion starts in some areas after 4 days and the skin peels off by the 6th day
- The skin will be pink and flesh colored for the next 7–10 days
- Hyperpigmentation starts in another 7 days and completely pigments sometimes with residual hypopigmentation and some areas of hyperpigmentation.

Delayed Complications

Hyperpigmentation/Hypopigmentation

Hyper- and hypopigmentation can occur after 4 weeks of the IPL treatment without any signs of burns or erosion.

Hyperpigmentation can occur mainly due to sun exposure following the treatment. Use of sunscreens postprocedure should be strictly followed. Use of triple combination for 7–10 days with only 1 hour contact and wash would rectify this complications.

Hypopigmentation is less common compared to hyperpigmentation, and usually occurs with higher energy used during the procedure and in some cases some patients have a tendency to hypopigment following treatment. This complication resolves by itself in 2–3 months or targeted phototherapy can be advised to hasten the pigmentation process. Two to three treatments of targeted phototherapy is sufficient (Figure 1).

Potential Infections

Bacterial infections following erosions due to aggressive treatments is common, antibacterial cream applied twice a day would suffice.

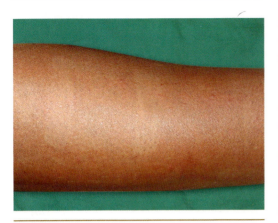

Figure 1: Showing area of hypopigmentation. The reason for this bands of hypopigmented areas is the difference in contact cooling time between shots.

Some patients develop herpes simplex infection, it is commonly seen when the upper lip hair removal is done. A course of oral acyclovir with topical ointment is needed in such cases.

Scars and Keloids

Scars and keloids are uncommon complications of IPL, however they do occur due to various reasons:

- Hyperpigmentation in the hair bearing areas
- Repeated plucking or tweezing of unwanted hairs can make the area hyperkeratotic with hyperpigmentation
- Patient applying hair dye, mascara, or any black pigment products to color the gray hairs. The black pigment gets absorbed in the upper layers of the epidermis.

Any of these reasons can results in unwanted burns to the skin which can be deep enough to cause scars or keloids in susceptible individuals when skin lightening or hair removal is done.

In case hyperpigmentation is present near the area decided for hair removal, advice the patient to use a Kligman regimen cream.

Patient has to apply for a contact period of 1 hour daily, starting 10 days before the procedure. This would lighten the pigment and make the skin less susceptible to burns.

Always ask the patient any history of hair dye or coloring near the area where you have planned for skin lightening or hair removal.

Paradoxical Hair Growth

Two explanations have been offered for paradoxical hair growth.[6] First, suboptimal fluences may activate dormant hair follicles in surrounding untreated areas leading to hair growth. Second, direct light synchronized hair growth cycles by first damaging exposed anagen follicles.

Next, a new follicular rhythm in unexposed dormant hair follicles in untreated areas close to the treated ones is established. Since hair growth in surrounding areas is now synchronized, overall hair density appears to be greater compared to previous asynchronous hair growth.

Dark skin (types III–V) may be a risk factor for the paradoxical effect.[7] A trend for the paradoxical effect to occur in darker skin phototypes (IV) compared to unaffected subjects was observed.

Ways to prevent paradoxical hair growth are:
- Use of sufficient fluence or avoiding suboptimal energy
- Double pass technique
- Treating additional areas slightly further from the decided areas
- Use of ice pack and firing in the central area of the cooled zone (Figure 2).

❑ CASE DISCUSSIONS

Case 1 (Figure 3)

A. The patient had come for removal of moustache. He wanted it to be removed because he was noticing gray hairs and wanted to it to be removed before they all turn gray. After counseling the patient not to do it, he still opted for hair removal

B. The patient came after 4 days with severe erosion and ulcerations which the authors have never encountered. When reason for the complications was pondered on,

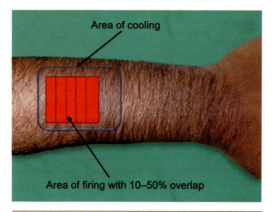

Figure 2: Showing area to be cooled and the placement of the intense pulsed light probe with overlap.

it was understood that the patients had applied hair dye to the moustache 3 days prior to the procedure. It was a mistake on the authors part not to ask the patient the particular history though it is not routinely asked for

C. Wounds healed by secondary intension, carbon dioxide fraxel with kenacort injection for the hypertrophic scar was to minimize the damage

D. The patient came back after 3 months with residual scarring and 40% reduction in hair, still wanting to complete the procedure.

Case 2

Hair removal near the vermillion border should not be attempted with IPL. Diode or long pulsed neodymium-doped yttrium aluminum garnet would be better choice.

When the vermillion border is crossed with the IPL probe, it causes burns because of the darker color of the lips and results

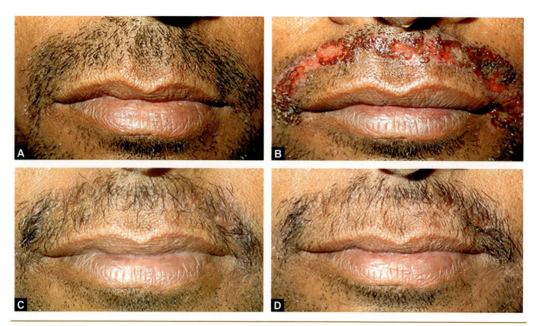

Figure 3: A, 0 day; **B,** 4 days post op; **C,** 6 weeks post op; **D,** 3 months post op.

in hypopigmentation (Figure 4). Targeted phototherapy or PUVAsol would help in faster repigmentation.

Case 3

Skipped areas of hair removal is common in the neck area (Figure 5). Most common reason being the position of the operator. When doing the chin, the operator should approach from the side of the patient to have proper visibility of the area being treated. Overlap is essential to prevent this mistake.

Also note the white hypopigmented dots in areas where previous hairs were present,

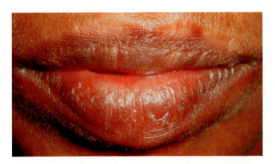

Figure 4: Crossing of vermillion border resulting in hypopigmentation.

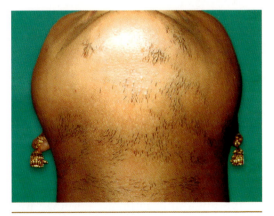

Figure 5: Skipped areas.

it denotes effective damage to the treated hairs which is seen in some cases. The hypopigmentation usually resolves in 3–6 weeks.

Case 4 (Figure 6)

Paradoxical hair growth is seen after 13 months in areas shown by the arrow, eight treatments of IPL was performed at an interval of 4–8 weeks.

Good clearance of hair from the chin and side burns (circled area) but new hairs because of paradoxical hair growth are seen in the cheek. This was common in 2005 when the authors first started using IPL.

Now using the techniques mentioned previously, with the cooling pad, this complications is greatly prevented.

Case 5 (Figure 7)

Usually, the flash lamp loses its optimum output after 8,000 fires (depending on the manufacturer). To compensate for the loss, 3–5 J/cm^2 is given more than the desired energy. Once the flash lamp is changed, one has to start from the normal energy. In this case, the flash lamp of the IPL had been changed because the previous flash lamp had completed its total fires. However the energy used was slightly higher leading to superficial burns. This is one of the most common complications seen with IPL.

A. The burn on the lip occurred when the patient sneezed and the crystal slipped over the lip at the time of firing. This is common when doing upper lip, when the cool tip of the crystal touches the nostrils or the smell of burnt hair, some patients have a tendency to sneeze so one has to be aware of that

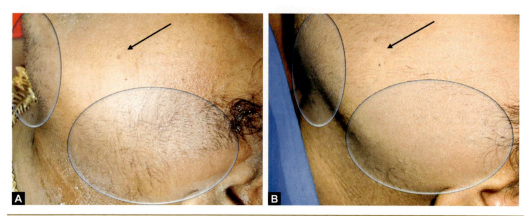

Figure 6: A, Intense pulsed light was done on the circled areas; **B,** good clearance after eight sessions in the treated areas but paradoxical hair growth in the nontreated areas.

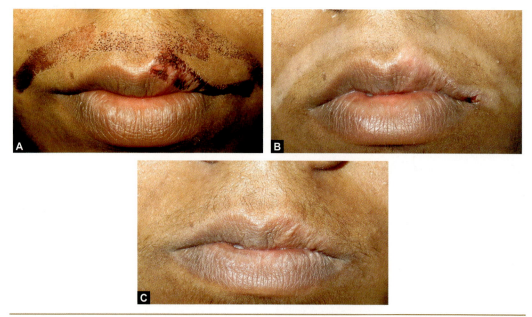

Figure 7: A, Epidermolysis due to excess energy and slipping of the probe while firing; **B,** 7 days post op; **C,** complete recovery in 6 weeks.

B. Epidermal growth factor was applied immediately after the procedure and the Figure 7B shows healing with hypopigmentation in one week

C. Complete healing was seen when the patient came for the next session. No damage to texture of the lip.

Case 6 (Figure 8)

- This patient developed milia formation and folliculitis 1 month post IPL for hair removal
- Carbon dioxide laser was used to open the milia and antibiotic coverage was given. Pyruvic peel was done after 3 weeks

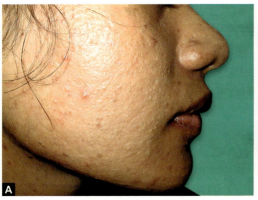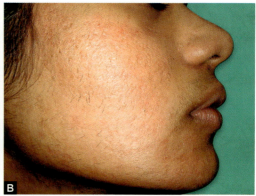

Figure 8: **A,** Milia formation following hair removal; **B,** treated with carbon dioxide laser and pyruvic acid peel.

to reduce the acneiform eruptions and improve the skin texture post laser.

Case 7 (Figure 9)

- In this case, the operator had forgotten to use the filter for hair removal which resulted in blistering and epidermolysis
- Note the mistake of randomly placing the handpiece and not overlapping the shots
- Always check the filter and light emitted before making the first shot
- Epidermal growth factor will be of great help in this complication.

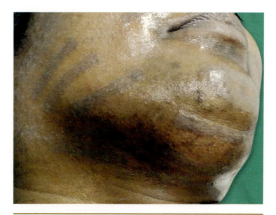

Figure 9: Burns and epidermolysis following failure to use a filter.

Case 8 (Figure 10)

A. Hemangioma since birth
B. In case of hemangioma, 560 nm filter is used to target deeper and larger vessels, but the target is large so energy in excess of 45 J/cm² (normally 23–28 J/cm² is enough to activate the yellow filter 560 nm) was used to improve the outcome
C. This resulted in blistering and ulceration, which should occur when higher energy is used
D. This heals well because epidermal growth factor and good vasculature in 3 weeks

E. After eight sessions 6 weeks apart, there was good improvement with residual hyperpigmentation which can be tackled with a Q-switched neodymium-doped yttrium aluminum garnet laser
F. Since higher energy was used more than the required energy for that particular filter, the other wavelengths after 560 nm, namely, 585, 690, and 755 nm all were also activated because it had reached sufficient fluence. This resulted hair removal from the treated areas which is marked by the blue rectangle for comparison.

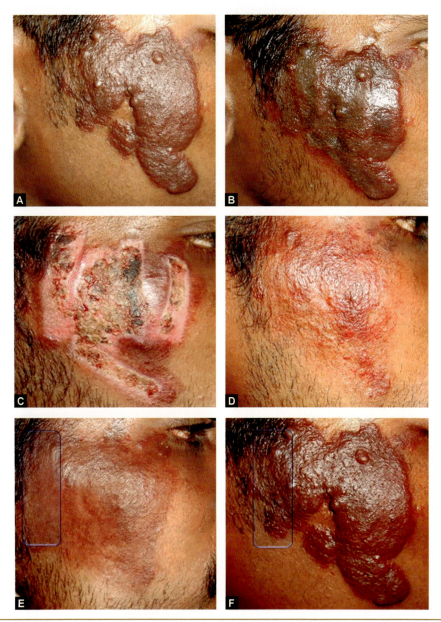

Figure 10: Treatment of hemangioma which resulted in hair reduction due to use of increased energy to treat hemangioma which resulted in activation the wavelengths 640–755 nm.

❏ ADDITIONAL INFORMATION

- Specific indications for each filter, and the targeting chromophore should be understood before attempting IPL (Table 2)

- When patient comes for subsequent treatments, an increase of 1–2 J can be given above the previous treatment. The reason being the skin lightens with subsequent treatments because there is

TABLE 2: Wavelength filters and their applications	
400–410 nm	Acne treatment
510–530 nm	Epidermal pigmentation, superficial vascular work skin rejuvenation
550–570 nm	Vascular work, acne, postacne redness, rosacea, skin rejuvenation
585–590 nm	Collagen remodeling, deeper and larger vascular lesions
640 nm	Collagen remodeling, hair removal in type I and II
690 nm	Hair removal in type III and IV
755 nm	Hair removal in type V and VI

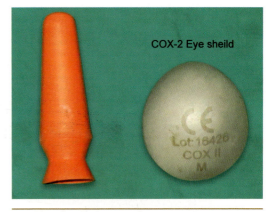

Figure 11: COX-2 eye shield.

reduction in melanin laden keratinocytes and patient has developed the habit of applying sunscreens postprocedure
- When contact ultrasound gel is used, see that it is transparent without any impurities. When IPL is used, the gel becomes opaque after 2–3 shots and there is fragments of hair embedded in the gel. This prevents the transmission of the light into the skin, so after every 2–3 shots clean the handpiece and apply new gel to next area
- Eye protection for both the patient and the operator is essential. Use of a saline soaked gauze over eyes before putting on the patient glasses will prevent any unwanted flash of light into the patient eyes. When IPL is done near the eye or eyebrow, use of an eye shield (COX-2) is definitely needed to prevent any damage to the eye (Figure 11). In case patient feels irritation or redness in eyes appears post-IPL, use of moxifloxacin with dexamethasone eye drops immediately after the procedure will alleviate the symptoms
- The green goggles filters the light from 190 to 1,800 nm, which is ideal for IPL (Figure 12), but the orange goggles filters between 190 and 540 nm and from 900 to 1,700 nm which is not suitable in hair

removal since it does not filter 640–755 nm. The wavelengths filtered by a particular goggles before using it should be noted
- The progression of wound healing following burns/blistering complications should be explained to the patient along with the time frame of how long it will take to bring the skin back to normal. The author did a test fire on his right forearm to find out the time frame for healing and these are findings (Figure 13):
  A. Three fires were done with 640 nm filter with three energies of 35, 38, and 40 J/cm^2 (left to right) without cooling
  B After 48 hours, there was slight erosion in the first and second strip of 35 and 38 J/cm^2 but blistering and peeling of skin in the third strip of 40 J/cm^2. Note the total epidermolysis revealing the upper dermis with pin point bleeding at the two corners but some amount of epidermis survived in the middle. Epidermal growth factor was applied only after 3 days, not immediately as suggested earlier
  C. After 15 days, the first two strips healed well, but the third strip showed hyperpigmentation because of per follicular pigmentation and complete epidermolysis

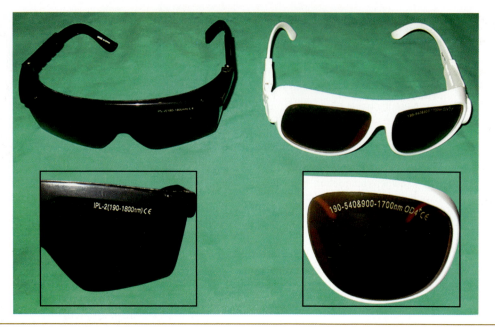

Figure 12: Look for the wavelength protection printed on the protective goggles before use.

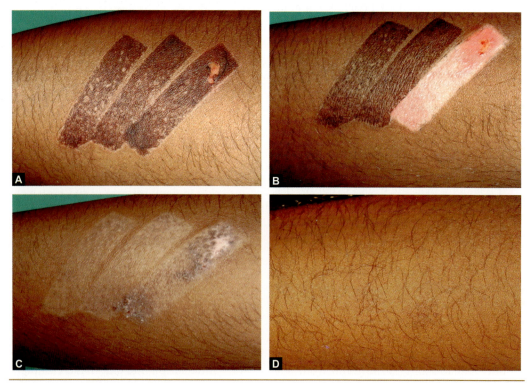

Figure 13: A, Immediate post op; **B,** 2 days post op; **C,** 15 days post op; **D,** 2 months post op.

D. After 2 months, almost complete recovery with mild hyperpigmentation. In this case, Kligman regimen was applied for 10 days in the third strip after complete healing to reduce the hyperpigmentation.

CONCLUSION

Before firing, one should always check if the correct filter is put on. Parameters should be adjusted according to patient and problem at hand. Proper filter should be chosen and the highest possible joules according to the patient's skin type should be used; hit hard at the first treatment. The placement of the handpiece, contact cooling time is different in different conditions, it has to be understood properly before attempting IPL. Use of skin lightening agents or treatment with 510–530 nm filter 2 weeks prior to doing 640 nm filter hair removal gives a better treatment outcome in darker skin types. Trimming the hair rather than shaving gives better results in IPL. Use of cooling pads in the nontreated areas in hair removal will prevent paradoxical hair growth. Overlapping shots with complete contact of skin with the crystal is essential in hair removal and rosacea. In other condition, random placing of the handpiece does not matter. Postprocedure complications like redness, epidermolysis, or blistering should be observed and treat accordingly. The authors advise use of epidermal growth factor postprocedure for 3 consecutive days. Botulinum toxin, even if injected immediately prior to IPL treatment, is not deactivated by the beam and is, therefore, not a contraindication to treatment.[8]

REFERENCES

1. Raulin C, Greve B, Grema H. IPL technology: a review. Lasers Surg Med. 2003;32(2):78-87.
2. Weiss RA, Sadick NS. Epidermal cooling crystal collar device for improved results and reduced side effects on leg telangiectasias using intense pulsed light. Dermatol Surg. 2000;26(11):1015-8.
3. Haedersdal M. Potential risks of non-physicians' use of lasers and intense pulsed light in dermatology. Ugeskr Laeger. 2005;167(43):4095-7.
4. Anderson RR, Parrish JA. Selective photothermolysis: precise microsurgery by selective absorption of pulsed radiation. Science. 1983;220:524-7.
5. Altshuler GB, Anderson RR, Manstein D, Zenzie HH, Smirnov MZ. Extended theory of selective photothermolysis. Lasers Surg Med. 2001;29(5):416-32.
6. Moreno-Arias GA, Castelo-Cranco C, Ferrando J. Paradoxical effect after IPL photoepilation. Dermatol Surg. 2002;28:1013-6.
7. Alajlan A, Shapiro J, Rivers J, MacDonald N, Wiggin J, Lui H. Paradoxical hypertrichosis after laser epilation. J Am Acad Dermatol. 2005;53:85-8.
8. Carruthers J, Carruthers A. The effect of full-face broadband light treatments alone and in combination with bilateral crow's feet Botulinum toxin type A chemodenervation. Dermatol Surg. 2004;30(3):355-66.

Complications of Hair Restoration Surgery

Vaishalee Kirane, Venkataram Mysore, Narendra Patwardhan

❏ INTRODUCTION

Complications in hair transplantation can be due to general or specific for hair restoration. Most complications are infrequent, minor, and can be avoided by proper technique. The commonest donor surgical complication is donor scarring and commonest recipient complication is postoperative edema.

Hair restoration surgery is usually a safe procedure and is associated with very few complications. However, as in all surgeries, complications can occur and the complications can be classified as below:

- Complications which are common to all surgeries such as lignocaine reactions, pain, infection, bleeding, keloids, etc.
- Others which are specific for hair transplantation[1-5]
  - Complications during anesthesia
  - Complications in donor area—intraoperative and postoperative
  - Complications in recipient area—intraoperative and postoperative
  - Poor results
  - Complications in special areas and situations
  - Complications of special techniques such as follicular unit extraction

The factors which may be responsible for these complications include:
- Unsuitable candidate selection, improper preoperative counseling, errors in preoperative assessment and inappropriate surgical planning
- Poor technique during donor area harvesting
- Errors during storage of the grafts
- Poor technique during recipient area implantation.

❏ GENERAL COMPLICATIONS

Adverse reactions to drugs may occur during anesthesia
- Adverse systemic reactions to local anesthetics fall into four categories: toxic, psychogenic, idiosyncratic, or allergic
- The overwhelming majority of adverse reactions to local anesthetics is psychogenic in nature and related to fear
- True immunologic reaction to a local anesthetic is rare
- All patients should be asked if they have received local anesthesia earlier
- Those who have not, should be tested with a test dose.

Other adverse reactions to drugs include drug induced gastritis to analgesics and antibiotics. These can be prevented by administration of antacids and H_2 blockers.

General intraoperative complications which may occur include tachycardia when tumescent fluid containing adrenaline is given. This is usually transient. However, in a cardiac compromised patient, this may pose a risk. Hence in all patients, particularly those who are above 40 years of age, an electrocardiogram and physician assessment is indicated.

Syncope: It is a complication which often occurs at the end of surgery, particularly if it is a long surgery. This may be due to pain, postural hypotension, xylocaine toxicity (poor hydration, hypoglycemia, etc.)

All these are avoidable by:
- Proper anesthesia and analgesia
- Making the patient sit before he gets up
- Minimizing xylocaine usage by completing surgery quickly
- Proper water, electrolytes, and nutrition balance
- Preoperative administration of clonidine 0.5 mg helps in prevention of syncope by its anticholinergic and analgesic activity (personal study).

Pain during Surgery and Postoperative Pain

Pain during surgery and postoperative pain are the commonest complication and is easily handled by proper surgical technique and use of analgesics. Factors which contribute to pain include wide strip, bleeding, wound tension, large sessions with inadequate anesthesia. Adequate postoperative analgesia can be prevented by:
- Paracetamol, codeine, and similar analgesics
- Postoperative administration of prednisolone which reduces wound edema.

Postoperative Hiccups

It is another rare but important complication as it can last up to 2–3 days. The cause is not known but may be due to stimulation of sensory divisions of C 2,3,4 nerves which also innervate diaphragm through phrenic nerve.[6]

❏ DONOR SITE COMPLICATIONS IN FOLLICULAR UNIT TRANSPLANTATION

Strip technique involves excision of a strip of skin followed by suturing. This is a step which is associated with most common problems as it is the step which needs proper surgical expertise.

Bleeding

Scalp being highly vascular, bleeding is expected. The possibility is more if the patient is on warfarin or any other anti-platelet drug.[7] After consulting with relevant physician such medicines need to be stopped at least 1 week before surgery. Bleeding can be prevented by adhering to few simple tips.

The various ways to prevent or treat it are:
- Tumescence to raise hair follicles away from underlying neurovascular plane
- Waiting for 10–15 minutes for tumescence to act
- Anxiety, if any, is alleviated by talking to the patient and calming him. Anxiolytics and sedatives are prescribed the night before and morning of surgery to decrease this risk
- Preoperative clonidine to allay anxiety and lower blood pressure
- Removing strip in parts, not in one piece
- Blood pressure is monitored and treated accordingly
- Avoiding deep incision-scoring superficially first followed by stretching the wound edges by a Haber spreader or skin hooks
- Proper surgical skill.

Once bleeding occurs, it needs to be controlled by pressure, using an artery forceps or electrocautery. As for as possible electrocautery should be avoided.

Folliculitis

Inflammation of one or more hair follicles can occur in donor area. While suturing, hair can get stuck in the suture line and lead to folliculitis. Pits can occur due to improper suturing. Folliculitis decalvans like recurring and persistent condition has also been reported, which becomes very chronic and distressing to the patient.[8]

Infection

It does not occur often in scalp surgery because of the high vascularity. Although prophylactic antibiotics are routinely administered, its value remains controversial. A study shows its value when administered just before surgery.[9] Infection may occur due to nonadherence to aseptic norms of surgery or lowered patient resistance. If infection does occur, appropriate antibiotics after sensitivity testing is necessary.[10] Lower risk of infections has been reported by treating nasal colonization of *Staphylo coccus aureus* by the application of mupirocin ointment and preoperative shampooing of scalp hair with use of chlorhexidine gluconate medicated soap the night before and the morning of surgery.[11,12] Septicemia has been reported after hair transplant.

Wound Dehiscence or Necrosis[13]

Wound dehiscence or necrosis of the donor wound site is a very unusual complication and mostly due to excessive removal of tissue of width more than 1.5 cm and wound closure under extreme tension. Overzealous use of cautery to achieve hemostasis will impair wound healing. Wound dehiscence is more common in elderly, those with vascular compromise and malnutrition. The author has seen a case where there was wound dehiscence in two patients after using monocryl, with formation of granulomatous tissue. Proper wound care, dressings, and antibiotics help heal the wound which may however take 2–4 weeks. The wound heals with a wider scar which may need subsequent grafting with hairs. Necrosis of the recipient area is much rarer and was seen when laser assisted holes were made, interfering with the circulation. Attentive evaluation for factors of tissue compromise like diabetics, smokers, and older age will help. The necrotic area is first debrided and scar excision done after healing takes place.

Numbness

It is usually transient and can occur because of transection of superficial sensory branches during donor strip excision.

Pain

Pain can result especially if donor wound is closed under extreme tension or due to damage to the underlying neurovascular supply. This is prevented by injecting sufficient tumescent solution of saline with 0.5% lidocaine/ bupivacaine and 1:50,000 epinephrine to raise the donor tissues and enabling cutting above the plane of the deeper neurovascular structures.[14]

Persistent Pain

Though rare, some patients complain of persistent pain for several weeks, possibly to development of neuropraxia and neuromas. Gabapentin, intralesional steroid injection are helpful in such cases.

Suture Extrusion

Suture extrusion rarely occurs.

Keloids

Keloids are rare on scalp. However, hypertrophic scarring can occur.

Donor Hair Effluvium

Donor hair effluvium or donor shock loss may occur particularly in post-auricular area, particularly after tight wound closure. It usually heals in few weeks but may cause great anxiety to the patient.

Donor Site Scars (Figure 1)

Donor site scarring occurs in all techniques used in HRS with the scars ranging from imperceptible to noticeable and very unsightly and disfiguring.

In strip excision technique of graft harvesting, a wide linear donor scar is the most feared consequence of modern HRS. This mainly results due to an increased tension on the donor wound closure in the occipital scalp area and mainly determined by the laxity of the occipital scalp skin. Asians in particular have a tendency for wider scarring.

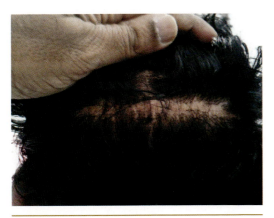

Figure 1: Donor site scarring.

Various preventive and corrective steps to avoid a wide unsightly donor scar are:[15]

- Scalp laxity exercises started 4 weeks prior to the surgery[16]
- Not extending the width of the donor strip to more than 1–1.5 cm, and closing the donor wound using sound surgical principles
- Good donor harvesting by skilled surgical technique and tumescence to raise from underlying neurovascular structures
- Double layer suturing
- Trichophytic closure method
- Minimizing the use of electrocautery to stop bleeding and instead applying compression for minimum 5–6 minutes will improve healing of the donor wound
- Corticosteroid like 3.33 mg/mL solution of triamcinolone acetonide mixed with bupivacaine 0.5% (prolongs the anesthetic effect) in dose of 5–6 mL is injected intralesional inferior to the closed wound immediately after
- Oral steroids in a tapering dose has also shown to decrease edema and wound tension.

❑ RECIPIENT AREA COMPLICATIONS

Poor Hair Line

A proper hairline in HRS is very important to give a natural frame to the face as onlookers visualize a person mainly from the front. The mid-scalp and the vertex play the next important role. Shapiro felt that proper selection and use of follicular units combined with artistry and skill provide surgeons with the tools to follow nature's lead in creating natural-appearing, soft hairlines while establishing the illusion of density.[17]

Several problems can occur due to improper frontal hair line like:

- Asymmetry: unnatural straight line hairlines with poor temporal angles is very common and reflect poor technique entirely. It is essential to design a natural, age-related proper hairline, taking efforts so as to avoid asymmetry. This can be done two-dimensionally with the help of mirror and three-dimensionally when the hairline is examined straight on. Ruler and laser guiding system additionally can be used to help plan an appropriate hairline by the starting surgeon who has not developed an eye for symmetry. Hairlines differ based on gender with female hairlines appear more rounded without the bitemporal recession occurring in males
- Cornrow plugs resulted in the time of the old punch grafting technique and are unaccepted in the modern follicular unit hair transplant method. They especially are exposed as the residual hair recedes and then necessitate correction. It can still occur if larger units are used for hair line
- Too low positioned hairline on the forehead and blunting of the temporal angles. The hairline should never be placed below a point 6 cm from the glabella which can result in dissatisfaction of the patient over time, especially in the case of evolving progressive hair loss behind the transplanted hairline.

Low Perceived Cosmetic Density and Unnatural Coverage

Low perceived cosmetic density and unnatural coverage of the bald area reflect errors in surgical and aesthetic judgment, performing procedures on noncandidate patients, surgical distribution of grafts that failed to consider the possibility of progressive hair loss in young patient of genetic pattern hair loss and failure to communicate successfully with patients

about realistic expectations also remain major problems even with latest follicular unit transplant technique. The surgeon needs to consider whether there will be sufficient projected donor hair to cover future hair loss.

Correction and repair of hair transplants require great skill and judgment. The focus is on creative aesthetic solutions to solve the supply/demand limitations inherent in most repairs. Corrective hair transplant procedure involves removal of the plugs partially leaving behind a few hairs which will look soft and natural, combining with scalp reduction surgery if needed and camouflage with transplanting additional follicular units using follicular unit extraction method either from the scalp occiput or body hairs to give further density.[18,19]

Recipient Area Edema (Figure 2)

This is common on 3–5th day of surgery, starting on the forehead and gradually spreading on to eyelids and nose. The precise relevance varies, but may occur in 3–8% of patients. The precise reason is not known, but several factors are thought to be responsible.
- Trauma of the surgery
- Large quantity of the tumescent solution injected in the recipient area. Intra-operative bleeding
- Gravity which pulls the fluid down

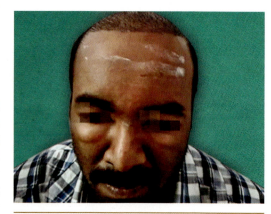

Figure 2: Recipient area edema.

- Lymphatic drainage of frontal scalp
- Loose donor skin, large sessions, elderly patients are more likely to experience it.

A prophylactic measure includes the use of short course of postoperative steroids. Injecting dilute steroid into the anterior scalp ring block can help to minimize the extent of postoperative edema. However, this may not obviate the possibility and occurrence of swelling mostly from the 3-5th day postoperative occurring on the forehead and in the periorbital area. An elastoplast band on the forehead at the end of surgery may also help. Abbassi solution was shown to prevent it. Reclining position for 24 hours though impractical may help. Ice packs used frequently once it develops, manual massage to push fluids to the sides are also useful.[20]

Postoperative Pustules (Figure 3)

Postoperative pustules which occur 1–3 months after surgery is related to presence of poorly dissected grafts and is related to graft dissection technique. It is sterile and usually heals by itself and may need drainage of pus.

Central Scalp Necrosis

Central scalp necrosis can occur after large sessions in elderly with vascular compromise. It is characterized by a dusky red discoloration of scalp followed by extensive crusting. It heals with central scar. While the exact cause is not known, it is postulated to the fact that central scalp receives comparatively less blood supply. Smoking, diabetes, actinic damage may predispose to the condition.[21]

Cobblestoning

Cobblestoning occurs from elevations and indentations of the scar tissue around the hair graft resulting in an unsightly uneven surface in the recipient area. This is when follicular unit grafts are implanted into too small a hole or at incorrect depth. Grafts should be placed only 1–2 mm above the surrounding surface to avoid this. The cobblestoning mostly improves with time or the scars may need to be excised. Postoperative pitting can also occur in recipient area (Figure 4).

Cysts

Cysts appear as small skin-colored swellings around the transplanted hair follicles which can become erythematous and painful. They result due to small grafts slipping under the skin or from piggybacking one graft on top of the other. Treatment consists of incising

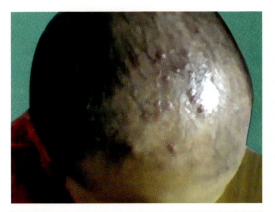

Figure 3: Post-operative pustules.

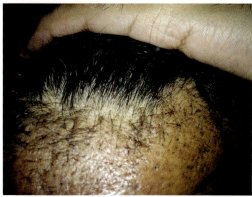

Figure 4: Recipient area pitting.

the cysts and expressing out the contents, warm compresses, or sometimes topical antibiotics.

Poor Hair Growth

Poor hair growth can occur when there is traumatic dissection of the hair grafts from the harvested strip or traumatic placement or dissection of the grafts. It can also be a result of poor quality donor hair like vellus hair which should be identified before surgery and thus such patient not selected for surgery. Patient should be counseled regarding the shedding of the transplanted hairs at around 6 weeks and the onset of new growth from 10 to 12 weeks with full growth achieved at 10–12 months. Decreased growth can also be due to factors like heavy smoking, diabetes is there proof that diabetes can lead to poor result and excessive sun damage to the scalp skin or sometimes due to nonspecific individual anatomic factors.

Temporary Hair Loss

Temporary hair loss called as shock loss is a kind of telogen effluvium of the surrounding hairs occurring due to the trauma of the surgery in 10–15% of males and more number in females. The patient can be forewarned about its possibility to alleviate anxiety or alarm. Use of topical minoxidil in males and females and oral finasteride only in males for at least 4–6 months prior to surgery can help to minimize this hair loss.

❏ TIPS AND PEARLS

- Thorough preoperative counseling regarding the benefits and limitations and risks of hair restoration surgery and recording in the medical chart goes a long way in preventing complications
- Selection of a suitable candidate for surgery, proper evaluation, and surgical planning of the recipient area

- Good design using sound surgical skills and techniques combined with artistry for hairline reconstruction and for high perceived midscalp or vertex cosmetic density and to record the same
- Avoid complications by meticulous preoperative assessment and good postoperative management
- Quality control for every step of the surgery should be on a continuous basis, improving whenever, and wherever possible.

❏ CONCLUSION

The most challenging part of starting hair restoration practice is not only the technique but also the lack of knowledge and experience required to avoid complications, recognize mistakes and correct them, and maintain consistency in quality. Since hair takes a minimum 6 months postoperatively to manifest substantive growth, the delay in learning from one's mistakes is sizeable. Unlike other surgeries, hair restoration involves a team of many assistants in charge of cutting and may be also placing grafts which can also contribute to complications or unfavourable results. Thus, success depends on technical expertise and quality control of both the surgeon and the team of assistants along with astute judgment in recognizing and correcting errors.

❏ REFERENCES

1. Loganathan E, Sarvajnamurthy S, Gorur D, Suresh DH, Siddaraju MN, Narasimhan RT. Complications of hair restoration surgery: a retrospective analysis. Int J Trichology. 2014;6(4):168-72.
2. Salanitri S, Gonçalves AJ, Helene A Jr, Lopes FH. Surgical complications in hair transplantation: a series of 533 procedures. Aesthet Surg J. 2009;29(1):72-6.
3. Konior RJ. Complications in hair-restoration surgery. Facial Plast Surg Clin North Am. 2013;21(3):505-20.
4. Perez-Meza D, Niedbalski R. Complications in hair restoration surgery. Oral Maxillofac Surg Clin North Am. 2009;21(1):119-48.

5. Lam SM. Complications in hair restoration. Facial Plast Surg Clin North Am. 2013;21:675-80.

6. Arnold J, Stough DB, Haber RS. Hair replacement. St. Louis: Mosby; 1996. pp. 332-4.

7. Otley CC, Fewkes JL, Frank W, Olbricht SM. Complications of cutaneous surgery in patients who are taking warfarin, aspirin, or non-steroidal anti-inflammatory drugs. Arch Dermatol. 1996;132:161-6.

8. Otberg N, Wu WY, Kang H, Martinka M, Alzolibani AA, Restrepo I, et al. Folliculitis decalvans developing 20 years after hair restoration surgery in punch grafts: case report. Dermatol Surg. 2009;35(11):1852-6.

9. Kaiser AB. Antimicrobial prophylaxis in surgery. N Engl J Med. 1986;315(18):1129-38.

10. Zoumalan RA, Rosenberg DB. Methicillin-resistant Staphylococcus aureus—positive surgical site infections in face-lift surgery. Arch Facial Plast Surg. 2008;10(2):116-23.

11. Van Rijn MM, Bode LG, Baak DA, Kluytmans JA, Vos MC. Reduced costs for Staphylococcus aureus carriers treated prophylactically with mupirocin and chlorhexidine in cardiothoracic and orthopaedic surgery. PLoS One. 2012;7(8).

12. Farjo N. Infection control and policy development in hair restoration. Hair Transplant Forum Int. 2008;18:141-4.

13. Karaçal N, Uralo lu M, Dindar T, Livao lu M. Necrosis of the donor site after hair restoration with follicular unit extraction (FUE): a case report. J Plast Reconstr Aesthet Surg. 2012;65(4):e87-9.

14. Wesley CK, Unger RH, Rosenberg M, Unger MA, Unger WP. Factors influencing postoperative hyperesthesia in hair restoration surgery. J Cosmet Dermatol. 2011;10(4):301-6.

15. Unger WP. Correction of cosmetic problems secondary to hair transplantation. In: Unger WP, Shapiro R, editors. Hair transplantation, 4th ed. New York: Marcel Decker; 2004. pp. 372-9, 475-80.

16. Mayer M, Pauls T. Scalp elasticity scale. Hair Transplant Forum Int. 2005;15:122-3.

17. Shapiro R. Principles and techniques used to create a natural hairline in surgical hair restoration. Facial Plast Surg Clin North Am. 2004;12(2):201-17.

18. Bernstein RM, Rassman WR, Rashid N, Shiell RC. The art of repair in surgical hair restoration part I: basic repair strategies. Dermatol Surg. 2002;28(9):783-94.

19. Vogel JE. Correcting problems in hair restoration surgery: an update. Facial Plast Surg Clin North Am. 2004;12(2):263-78.

20. Gholamali A, Sepideh P, Susan E. Hair transplantation: preventing postoperative Oedema. J Cutan Aesthet Surg. 2010;3(2):87-9.

21. Yildiz H, Ercan E, Alhan D, Sezgin M. Recipient site necrosis after tumescent infiltration with adrenaline in hair transplantation. Acta Dermatovenerol Croat. 201p;23(3):233-4.

Complications of Fillers

Malavika Kohli, Rajul Davda

☐ INTRODUCTION

The popularity of dermal fillers has grown in recent years because they offer rejuvenative and enhancing effects, previously only available through surgery at a lower cost and minimal downtime.

According to data from American Society of Plastic Surgeons, the percentage of minimally invasive cosmetic procedures is on the rise (Table 1 and Figure 1).

As public awareness and acceptance of dermal fillers grows, so does the size of the market with an estimated 160 products currently available worldwide from more than 50 companies.

TABLE 1: Upward trend in cosmetic procedures
15.6 million cosmetic procedures ▲ 3%
• 1.7 million cosmetic surgical procedures ▲ 1%
• 13.9 million cosmetic minimally-invasive procedures ▲ 4%

Increasingly, fillers are being used for volume replacement and enhancement procedures,[1] cheek and chin augmentation, tear trough filling, nose reshaping, mid-face volumization, lip enhancement, hand rejuvenation besides the usual indications of filling rhytides and folds, and correction of soft tissue loss due to disease or age.[2]

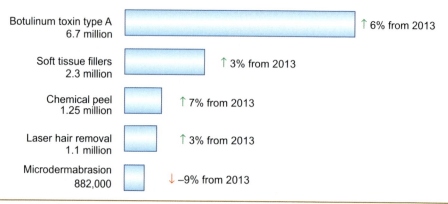

Figure 1: 2014 top five cosmetic minimally-invasive procedures.

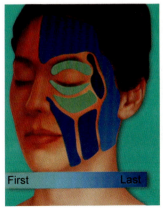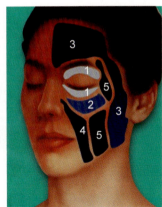

Figure 2: Aging fat.

As the indications and the number of procedures performed increase, the number of complications will likely also increase.

It is therefore necessary for the injector to understand facial anatomy, injection techniques, and the different properties of available fillers in order to reduce the risk of complications, improve patient outcomes and care for patients who have experienced adverse effects.

❑ PREPROCEDURE CARE

Know How the Face Ages

Though aging is a generalized phenomenon, the process of aging does not occur uniformly in all areas of the face. The subcutaneous fat of the face is not a single uniform layer but is compartmentalized.[3-5] Each individual compartment ages at a different pace in the same individual. Hence, we need to identify which fat compartment has changed first and the most and prioritize this area to maximize filler injection outcomes and enhancement.

In a younger patient, the orbital and superficial cheek fat pad are the first to get affected. This is why in Indian patients tear trough correction is the most common request,

another being to restore the "freshness" which can start in someone as young as 35 years of age (Figure 2).

Know Your Filler Product and Its Specifics

There are a host of fillers now available in India. By far the most popular fillers are the hyaluronic acid (HA) based ones. There is a spectrum of HA fillers and hence, it is imperative to know each ones specifics, their 'G' prime, particles per milligram, cross-linking, monophasic or biphasic nature, presence of any additive like lignocaine, and their shelf life.

❑ CATEGORIES OF DERMAL FILLERS

There are several methods of categorizing dermal fillers (Flowchart 1).

For a discussion of dermal filler complication, it is perhaps most useful to categorize in terms of biodegradable versus nonbiodegradable.

Hyaluronic acid fillers are the most widely used biodegradable fillers[6,7] and generally have effects lasting 6–18 months. Hyaluronic acids are linear polymeric dimers of N-acetyl glucosamine and gluuronic acid.

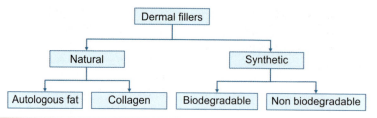

Flowchart 1: Categorization of dermal filler.

Various HAs have different properties depending on the proprietary methods used to cross link their dimers, their degree and method of chain cross linking, the uniformity and the size of their particles and their concentration. These characteristics have significant impact on the clinical effects of these products.

Increased cross linking and concentration increases the viscosity and elasticity and the resistance to degradation by native hyaluronidase.

Various technologies like NASH, hylacross, Vy cross, and CPA are cross linking techniques and these are company specific. One needs to know these as an injector from the ease of injection point of view and longevity of the product. The accompanying needles that are provided with each individual filler also enhance the ease of injection and therefore the injector's skill.

The authors experience is that as one injects more and gains more experience and confidence these cross linking techniques are almost comparable in the properties they lend to the filler material.

Increased concentration and large particle size will increase the hydrophilic nature of the product and hence cause more tissue swelling after the procedure. Different HAs have varying degrees of hardness (G'), which will influence their suitability for a particular procedure. In general, the greater the G' of the product the deeper it should be injected.

It should be noted that while more concentrated products with greater cross linkage have a longer duration of effect, they could also increase the possibility of hypersensitive reactions.

Know the Technique

There are various methods of injecting filler. Most popular is the linear threading method, either retrograde or ante grade. It is advisable that the beginners start with this technique than other techniques like the depot or fern method, which need more expertise with ease of flow of product as it can be associated with lumps, if given inappropriately.

Historically, fillers were injected through sharp needles of various gauges depending on the viscosity of the product. Cannulas came out a little over 5 years and injecting through a cannula became a rage as it caused less bruising and one could traverse difficult areas with ease (Table 2).

TABLE 2: Pros and cons of needle versus cannula technique	
Needle	**Cannula**
Short length	Long length
Sharp	Blunt
Multiple entry points required	Single entry point
More traumatic	Less traumatic
More bruising	Less bruising
Placement of material maybe uneven	Uniform placement of product

However, the present status is that there are equal number of proponents for cannula and needle users and the choice really depends on the injectors comfort level and experience.

Assess the Patient

- Know the psyche of the patient: it is important to allay fears of any kind that the patient may have before starting the procedure. A patient with unrealistic expectations may always be dissatisfied
- Medical illness: risk of bruising is more when patients have bleeding disorders, uncontrolled hypertension, or are on blood thinners like aspirin, clopidogrel, warfarin.

Documentation

- Obtain informed consent
- Document the findings by taking well focused and standardized pre- and post-treatment photographs. Encourage the patient to animate so one can observe for their expressions, volume loss, and any asymmetry between the two sides
- Discuss the cost of the treatment.

Dermal Filler Complications: Avoidance and Treatment

All fillers are associated with a risk of both short and long duration complications. While most adverse reactions are mild and transient, one needs to be aware of the more infrequently but serious adverse events which may potentially leave patients with long-lasting functional and aesthetic deficits. Some reactions occur immediately post-treatment whereas some have delayed onset.

Type of adverse events by time of onset are illustrated in table 3.

TABLE 3: Complications	
Early	**Late**
• Erythema	• Granuloma
• Edema	• Migration
• Ecchymosis, bruising	• Hypertrophic scar
• Tyndall effect	• Telangiectasia
• Lump, nodule	• Skin compromise
• Vascular compromise	• Infection, biofilm
• Skin necrosis	
• Infection, biofilm	

Early

Edema and Erythema

Swelling may develop at the time of injection and it usually resolves spontaneously. Postprocedure erythema is usually transient (Figure 3), however, if erythema lasts for several days one should rule out infection by checking for accompanying local signs of inflammation and feeling of malaise. If not then consider the possibility of a hypersensitivity reaction.

Management

- Ice application and gentle pressure helps to reduce the swelling
- Erythema can be managed by topical vitamin K creams,[8-9] topical arnica gel and cold compresses
- Anti-inflammatory, such as nonsteroidal anti-inflammatory drugs, serratiopeptidase, and oral anti histaminics, can help to resolve the swelling faster
- If the swelling persists and is accompanied with local signs of inflammation with or

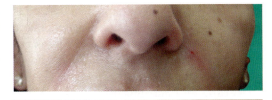

Figure 3: Transient erythema immediately after filler.

without malaise, one should empirically start oral antibiotics such as clarithromycin (500 mg) twice a day or ciprofloxacin (750 mg) twice a day for 10–14 days

- If an infection is suspected at the very beginning avoid oral steroids and start antibiotics.

Antibody-mediated Edema (Angioedema)

Some patients may develop hypersensitivity to injected products due to an immunoglobulin E-mediated immune response (type I hypersensitivity reaction). This may occur after initial or repeated exposure. Angioedema occurs within hours of exposure. Reactions can be severe and can last for several weeks.[10] Edema may be confined to the injection sites, but may also be more generalized. An acute idiopathic allergic response can also occur in which no allergen can be identified; the reaction may be localized, or there may be acute generalized facial edema.

Management

Treatment of angioedema, whether of known cause or idiopathic, depends on the severity of the condition. In many cases, the swelling resolves spontaneously after a few hours or days. If mast-cell mediated, the swelling is short lived and responsive to antihistamines. For persistent edema or edema not responsive to antihistamines, oral prednisone is the mainstay of treatment (Flowchart 2).[11] The patient should be closely monitored to make sure the edema is not a result of an infectious etiology. Rapidly progressing angioedema is treated as a medical emergency because of the risk of airway obstruction. Chronic angioedema refers to episodes that last more than 6 weeks. These cases are often difficult to treat and have a variable response to medication.

Nonantibody-mediated (Delayed) Edema

Delayed hypersensitivity reactions are characterized by induration, erythema, and edema, and are mediated by T-lymphocytes rather than antibodies. They typically occur one day after injection, but may be seen as late as several weeks to months after injection and may persist for many months[12,13] (Figure 4). Delayed hypersensitivity reactions are nonresponsive to antihistamines. The allergen should be removed (Flowchart 2). In the case of HA, this will involve dissolving the filler material with hyaluronidase. Other more permanent fillers may require treatment with steroids until the filler resorbs, laser treatment, and/or extrusion.[14] Excision is a last resort. Symptoms should be controlled with the lowest possible dose of oral steroids (prednisone).

Malar Edema

Malar edema is an oft encountered and annoying complication that has been reported with all fillers when injected into the infra-orbital hollow and tear troughs. Malar bags may festoon more with inappropriately place filler product.

The infra-orbital hollow is the area bounded by the medial canthus medially, the lateral canthus laterally, and the inferior border of the orbicularis oculi under which lies the infra-orbital bony rim. This region is particularly susceptible to adverse events (Figures 5 to 7). Malar edema after dermal filler injection arises because the malar septum, a band of connective tissue divides the superficial suborbicularis oculi fat into a superficial and deep compartment. The superficial compartment has compromised lymphatic drainage, while the lymphatic drainage of the deep compartment is contiguous with the cheek drainage.[15] Injection

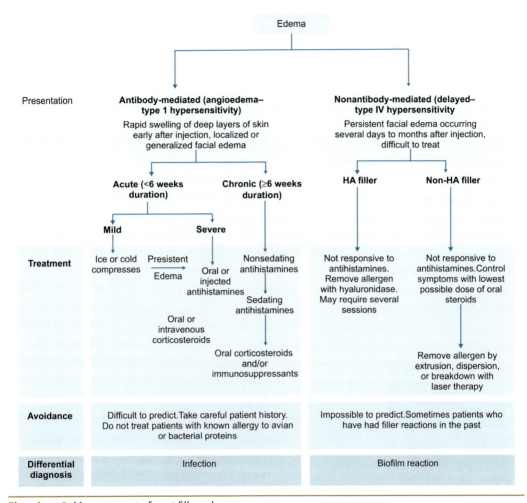

Flowchart 2: Management of post filler edema

HA, hyaluronic acid.

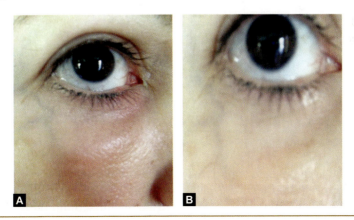

Figure 4: Local hypersensitivity reaction to product.

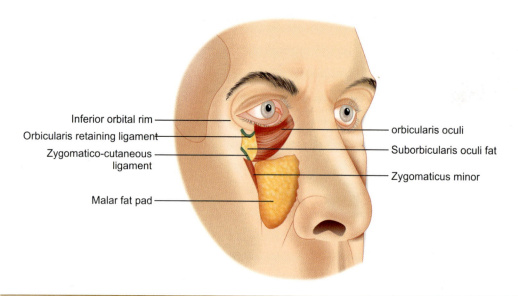

Figure 5: Anatomical position of suborbicularis oculi fat.

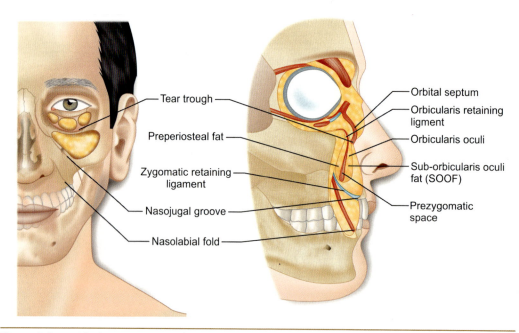

Figure 6: Anatomical structures contributing to malar bag formation.

of fillers superficial to the malar septum may augment the impermeable barrier of the malar septum, further impeding lymphatic drainage and resulting in fluid accumulation and malar edema.[16] Fillers injected superficial or deep to the malar septum may also cause edema

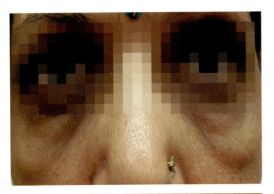

Figure 7: Preexisting malar bags.

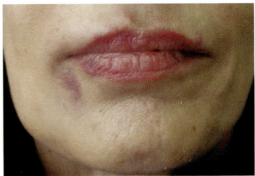

Figure 8: Bruising.

by direct pressure on the lymphatics when injection volumes are too large. In addition, as the viscosity or G' of the filler increases, the lifting force also increases, and the lymphatics may be more compressed. Some patients demonstrate malar edema without filler treatment, demonstrating existing lymphatic compromise. Malar edema, post-injection is likely related to the volume of injectable, its depth of injection, the physical qualities of the injectable, and the patient's degree of pre-existing lymphatic compromise.

Skin Discoloration

Ecchymosis and Bruising

One should look for vessels before injecting to avoid this complication. However, bruising may be inadvertent complication despite keen observation and anatomical variation and resolves spontaneously by 7 days (Figure 8).

Refining the Technique

It has been observed that bruising occurs more frequently when the filler is laid down by fanning and threading techniques. Less bruising is likely to occur when it is laid down as a depot in the preperiosteal level.[17]

The tear trough area is particularly treacherous. Using a sharp needle will always

have a higher chance of bruising, however thinner gauge cannulas such as numbers 27 and 30 are sharp and can produce equally bad bruising.

If the traumatized vessel is superficial, the bruising settles in 7–10 days, if however a deeper vessel is hit, the authors have come across a couple of cases where the bruising has lasted for several months (Figure 9). This is why it is advocated to not fill directly in the mid zone area of the infraorbital rim from wherein emerge the infraorbital vessels from the infraorbital foramen.

Management

Cold compresses, vitamin K creams and low intensity intense pulse light sessions every few days help in faster resolution.

Tyndall Phenomenon

A bluish hue may occur as a result of inappropriately placed and chosen HA filler. This is known as a Tyndall effect, which is a result of scattering of light by particles in suspension.[11] Most frequently, it is seen in the tear trough area and hence the dictum is to place the filler deep and supra periosteally in the peri-orbital rim irrespective of the product/needle or cannula.

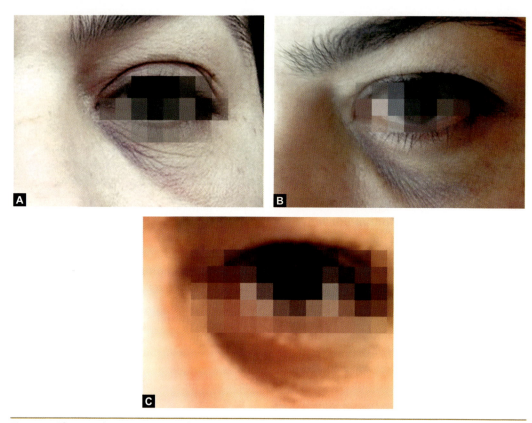

Figure 9: The treacherous tear trough: **A,** 2 days postprocedure; **B,** 2 months postprocedure; **C,** 6 months postprocedure.

Management

Hyaluronidase should be the initial approach to treatment. For HAs that are less susceptible to hyaluronidase because of high degree of cross linking or large particulate size, multiple treatments and larger volumes may be necessary. Incision and expression of the unwanted superficial filler can also be done.[18,19]

Lumps, Nodules

These appear as cystic, sclerotic, or edematous well-defined palpable lesions which occur either from:

- Injections in areas of thin soft tissue coverage (Figures 10 and 11; Table 5)
- Superficial injections (Figure 12)
- Injection of too much material.
- Clumping of material or dislocation from movement of muscles in hyperkinetic areas[20-22] (Figure 13).

Hyaluronic acid products are preferred in the high-risk areas (lips, periorbital, and nasojugal) as these irregularities can easily be resolved using hyaluronidase.

Management

In case of a cystic nodule is a simple puncture (incision and drainage) (Figures 13 to 18).

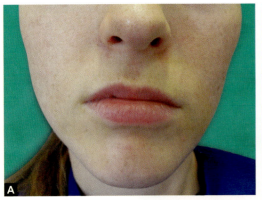
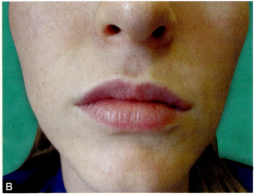
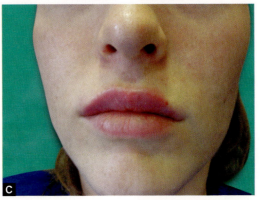

Figure 10: Sequence of events: **A,** Before; **B,** after; **C,** touch up after 15 days.

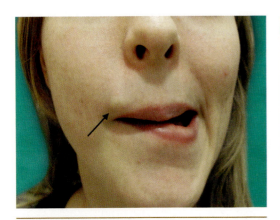

Figure 11: After injection nodule.

TABLE 5: Causes of lumps/nodules

- Placement of material—too superficial
- Excess material
- Viscosity of the material
- Displacement of material when placed in hyperkinetic muscle
- Granuloma formation
- Placement of material—too superficial

If it is a sclerosing type of nodule (occurs more frequently with semi-permanent filler) then direct excision will be required or observe until the product is absorbed.[23-26] They may also respond to intralesional steroids provided there is no infection.

Measures to avoid visibility of injected filler is to place the material in the correct tissue plane according to its viscosity, as specified by the company. It could be intradermal, subdermal, or supraperiosteal plane. Over massaging postprocedure may not help; a review after 48 hours or 7 days later, with a gentle massage may mold the material better.

Infection, Erythematous Nodule

As with any other invasive procedure, soft tissue filler injections too can cause infections. This can be completely avoided by taking necessary aseptic precautions and keeping the area to be treated completely sterile.

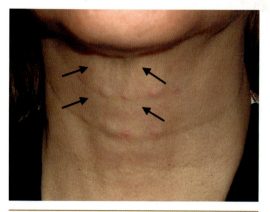

Figure 12: Superficial placement of hydrating filler causing a lumpy bumpy appearance. Correct placement is in the mid dermis.

Hair should be washed the morning of the procedure and should be completely off the face and banded and capped. The edge of the hairline should be sterilized, patient should be instructed to avoid touching the face while the treatment is going on, etc. are some of the measures besides the standard surgical sterilization procedures that one needs to undertake.

Excessive handling and too many handlers of the products and needles and cannulas should be avoided.

What the authors follow is to keep an alcohol swab in one hand and swipe it across the skin over each new area that has to be injected.

If single abscess gets formed, most likely contamination of skin occurred through the injection. If multiple abscesses are formed, there is a likelihood of contamination of the syringe prior to the injection.

For fluctuant abscesses, abscess culture with appropriate antibiotics are necessary along with incision and drainage.

For nonfluctuant abscesses, antibiotics are the first line of treatment. Oral steroids are often resorted to rapidly reduce edema but should be avoided as far as possible. Treatment algorithm is given in flowchart 3.[11]

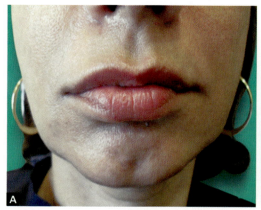
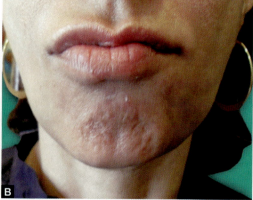

Figure 13: Lumps and bumps on chin due to placement of product under hyperkinetic mentalis.

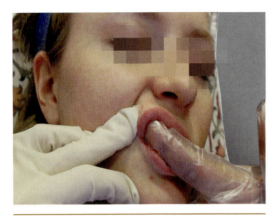

Figure 14: Extraction using 18 G needle to make a puncture and remove the hyaluronic acid.

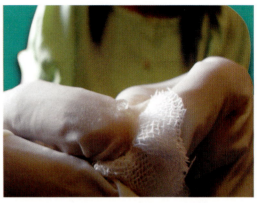

Figure 15: Extracted uninfected hyaluronic acid material.

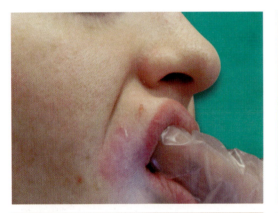

Figure 16: After removal.

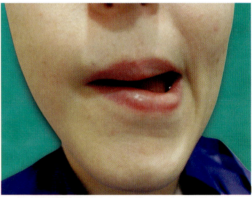

Figure 17: Two weeks after removal.

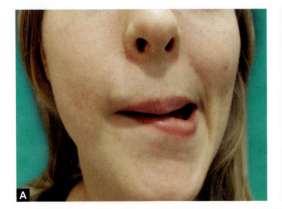

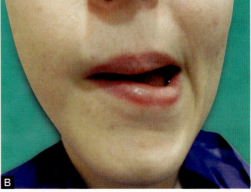

Figure 18: After 2 weeks of removing the extra material: **A,** Before; **B,** after.

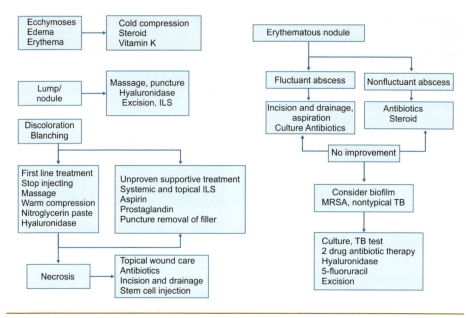

Flowchart 3: Algorithm to manage early complications.

ILS, intralesional steroids; MRSA, methicillin resistant *Staphylococcus aureus*; TB, tuberculosis.

In the early stages of treatment, hyaluronidase should not be used to avoid the risk of spreading the infected material in the surrounding tissues and a good course of oral antibiotics should be instituted.

If these treatments fail, one should suspect biofilm, methicillin-resistant *Staphylococcus aureus* or an atypical tuberculosis infection

Herpetic Outbreak

Dermal filler injections can lead to reactivation of herpes virus infections. If the treatment is targeting the lips or mouth area and the individual has a history of cold sores, prophylactic treatment with valaciclovir (500 mg twice daily for 3–5 days) can be started prior to injection to reduce the likelihood of this occurring (Figure 19). If supra-infection occurs, the patient should be treated with appropriate antibiotics. The majority of herpetic recurrences occur in the perioral area, nasal mucosa, and mucosa of the hard palate.

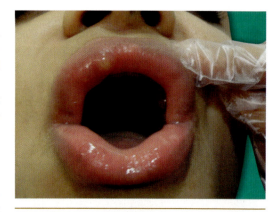

Figure 19: Lip augmentation done 5 years ago.

Vascular Compromise

Events related to vascular compromise should be handled as a medical emergency. These may occur as immediate or delayed events and are highly likely to result in permanent sequelae.

They can occur from:

• Intravascular embolism of injected material

- External compression of the adjacent vasculature secondary to the hydrophilic properties of the product[8]

This is especially true when too big a quantity of the filler product has been injected or the injection itself has been too fast.

All injectors should have a thorough knowledge of facial vasculature (both arteries and veins) to avoid inadvertent injections of the angular, dorsal nasal, labial, or supratrochlear artery as they are most likely to cause necrosis (Figure 20).[27,28]

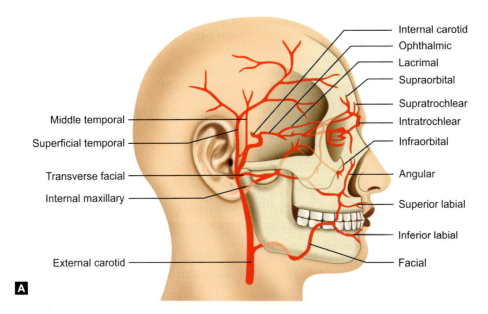

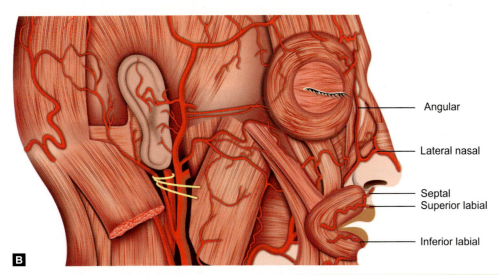

Figure 20: Arteries of the face.

Signs of Tissue Necrosis

Pathophysiology of vascular occlusion begins with immediate changes that are visible in the area of the skin overlying the injected vessel. Initial blanching of the skin may or may not occur. Delayed blanching can be seen a couple of hours later and one may get an unexpected communication from the patient.

If one notices blanching during the procedure immediately stop injecting; more so if it is accompanied by severe pain. Mottled discoloration called livedo reticularis may follow soon which is a sign of ischemia.

The resulting ischemia produces a dusky discoloration that is associated with a sluggish or absent capillary refill. The final stage of vascular compromise is skin necrosis which may occur a few days later.

The authors suggest that while injecting the above mentioned areas, the injector should be keenly observant and in tune with the patient. The authors would further suggest that the injections should be slow and controlled with just enough quantity of product.

However, anatomical variations in vascular architecture may spring up an odd event despite all care. Therefore, when injecting the pyriform fossa—the injection should either be intradermal or supraperiosteally. Stay intradermal in your depth when injecting the static glabellar lines. One may accidently injure the dorsal nasal artery while injecting the tear trough, if one goes too close to the medial canthus. This is especially true while using cannulas. It is best to avoid 27 and 30 number gauge cannulas while doing the tear trough.

Retinal Artery Occlusion

This is a rare event that occurs when dermal fillers enter into one of the distal branches of ophthalmic artery[29] after an inadvertent intra-arterial injection. These include the angular artery, zygomatico temporal, zygomatico facial, and dorsal nasal arteries, supratrochlear and supraorbital.

It is usually encountered while performing a medical rhinoplasty using fillers.[30-32] This could occur with a needle or a cannula.

Immediate blurring or loss of vision may occur.[33] Immediate and unlimited use of hyaluronidase should be employed to reverse or prevent blindness. Prompt consultation with ophthalmologist is crucial. Intraocular hyaluronidase has also been advocated.

Management

Vascular compromise is a medical emergency. Stop injecting and prioritize restoring the blood circulation to compromised area as timely intervention in the next crucial few minutes may help to avoid a catastrophe.

Injection should be stopped and area of injection should be massaged as well as warm compresses applied to increase vasodilatation.[8,34,35] Cold compresses should not be applied as it will worsen the vasoconstriction.

Nitroglycerin paste can also be used for vasodilatation. Although aspirin and intravenous prostaglandins have been suggested, their efficacy has not been proven.[36]

Hyaluronidase should be used to dissolve the product, facilitate blood flow, and promote vasodilation. Ideally, hyaluronidase should be preprepared and by ones side. Dayan et al.[37] have suggested the use of hyaluronidase in all cases of vascular compromise independent of the filler type.

It is advised to inject hyaluronidase not only in the areas where filler has been injected but also wherever one can see pallor, livedo reticularis, dusky erythema, and where the patient complains of pain. Anywhere from 1,500 to 15,000 units of hyaluronidase can be used to save a situation.

The patient should be asked to stay back and observed for at least 2–3 hours before one allows them to leave. During that time, one may need to inject some more hyaluronidase if the pallor/pain does not pass off.

It is important to make yourself and the entire team completely accessible at all times by providing hotline and emergency numbers. Encourage patients to send photographs electronically if they live far and call for a follow-up visit the next morning to reevaluate reversal of the compromised vasculature or to reassess the severity of the sequelae such as dusky erythema or signs of necrosis if any.

In Case of Necrosis

Antibiotics and wound management strategies to minimize scarring maybe required. If hyperbaric oxygen facilities are available, it should be administered to help survival of compromised tissue.

Adipose derived stem cells promote angiogenic processes and help in wound healing however exact mechanisms are not yet out in the open (Figure 21).[38]

Granuloma and Biofilm

Granulomas represent a type IV hypersensitivity reaction to injected foreign

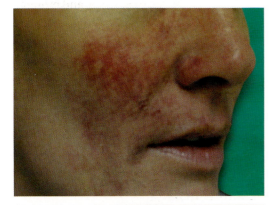

Figure 21: Vascular complications.

Courtesy: Dr Rungsima Wanitphakdeedecha.

material. Their incidence ranges from 0.01 to 14% according to the different chemical nature of fillers used[39]

They may develop as a delayed complication months or years after filler injection[40,41] and should be distinguished from early implant nodules, which usually develop 2–4 weeks after the injection.

Clinically, they are characterized by progressive development of papules, nodules, plaques with or without ulceration, and any material expressed is culture negative. The lesions tend to become firmer over time due to fibrosis and may lead to retracted, disfiguring scars.

The pathogenesis of these granulomatous reactions has been linked to the following possibilities:

- Hypersensitivity reactions
- Impurity of microimplants
- Bad technique
- Temporal combination—this refers to the use of different fillers at different times, often in patients who become addicted to multiple cosmetic injections sometimes performed by different injectors unaware of previous implants (Figure 22).[42]

Histopathology is very useful not only to achieve a diagnosis of granuloma induced by fillers but also to identify the type of microimplant, as the particular configuration of the vacuoles and cystic structures inside the granulomas reflects the shape of the injected implants particles.[43-47]

Permanent fillers carry a higher risk of granulomatous reactions. Although not common, biodegradable/resorbable fillers are also capable of inducing granulomatous reactions.

Management

First steps include identification of the injected material and exclusion of an infection. These are followed, in case of a HA filler granuloma, by intralesional hyaluronidase injection, and in case of all the other filling materials by an intralesional corticosteroids injection.[42]

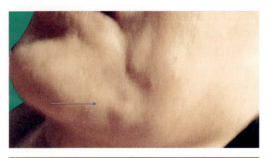

Figure 22: Granuloma/biofilm formation.

Patients with lesions unresponsive to steroids alone will benefit with the addition of 5-fluorouracil (5-FU) to the corticosteroids.

In case of repeated failure of other therapies, surgical excision is the treatment of choice.

Antimicrobial agents, especially minocycline or macrolides and fluoroquinolones, are often used successfully for the treatment of silicone granulomas due to their ability to inhibit bacterial growth and also to their direct immunosuppressive activity against granulomas.

Biofilms

Biofilms are accumulations of microorganisms within a self-developed matrix. They are irreversibly adherent to one another and to a variety of surfaces.[48]

In the biofilm, bacteria can safely avoid from immune defenses so antibiotics have no effect.[49]

Distinguishing inflammation due to a bacterial biofilm from a low-grade hypersensitivity reaction is difficult.

Persistent inflammatory conditions not showing improvement with other therapies and inflammatory nodules recurring after resolution may indicate a biofilm formation.

As they are usually culturally negative, these nodules were previously thought to be an allergic or a foreign body reaction to the filler substance. However, the technique of fluorescence *in situ* hybridization confirms an infective etiology.[50]

Preventive Measures

- Surgical sterilization of the entire face before injection (face should be completely devoid of makeup)
- Avoid injection through oral or nasal mucosa
- Avoid hydrophilic permanent materials
- Refrain from frequent injections
- Aggressive treatment of any after filler infection
- Indiscriminate use of oral and/or topical steroids.

Management

- Antibiotic therapy: this is the first line of treatment even if the culture is negative. It should be initiated with a broad spectrum agent like quinolone such as ciprofloxacin 500 mg bid and a macrolide such as clarithromycin 500 mg bid for 4–6 weeks
- Hyaluronidase should be used if the patient was injected with a HA filler
- Intralesional steroids should not be used before antibiotics as they can prolong the problem
- If long-term induration persists then treatment with 5-FU injection either alone or in combination with corticosteroid should be initiated and repeated every 2–4 weeks
- Laser lysis: intralesional subcutaneous introduction of an optic laser microfiber and the subsequent heat production results in a theoretical decrease of microbial counts on the biofilm and in liquefaction of the filler material
- Surgical excision should be the last resort.

Telangiectasia

Occasionally, permanent telangiectasia appear at the injection site and in patients

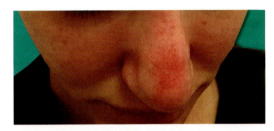

Figure 23: Telangiectasia.

with preexisting telangiectasia, injection of the filler worsens their appearance and size (Figure 23).

Management

Treatment with intense pulsed light or pulsed dye laser can be helpful.[20,21] Reduction of filler volume in the area may also help to reduce the pressure effect caused by more robust materials placed superficially.

Migration

Migration is thought to result from muscle or gravity induced displacement of the filler material.[20] It occurs when the filler is placed to superficially or in highly mobile anatomical areas like the lips, marionette line, or lid areas.

Patients should be warned to avoid massaging of the injected site and avoid strenuous exercise for 2–3 days after injection. For vocations where the patient needs to phonate (e.g., singers) a longer recovery time should be advised.

Management

Hyaluronic acid fillers can be tried to be massaged back into the desired area or hylased if that is not possible. Non-HA fillers can be treated with intralesional steroid and massage provided there are no signs of inflammation or infection.

Hypertrophic Scar

Superficial placement of fillers rarely resolves with permanent scarring consisting of extracellular components like collagen, fibroblasts, and small vessels.

Treatment can be attempted with a pulse dye laser or intralesional steroids or scar revision techniques and technology (Flowcharts 4 and 5).

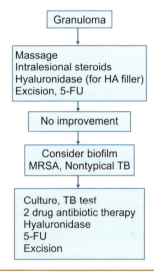

Flowchart 4: Algorithm for management of granuloma/biofilm.
5-FU, 5-fluorouracil; TB, tuberculosis; HA, hyaluronic acid; MRSA, methicillin resistant *Staphylococcus aureus*.

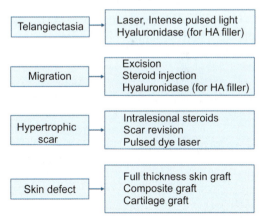

Flowchart 5: Management of late complications
HA, hyaluronic acid.

Hyaluronidase

Hyaluronidase is an enzyme that breaks down HA (hyaluronan) by cleaving glycoside bonds of HA and to some extent, other acid mucopolysaccharides of the connective tissue.[51]

In humans, six hyaluronidases have been identified (HYAL-1, -2, -3, -4, HYALP1, and PH-20).[52] Commercial formulations of hyaluronidase are of bovine (bovine testicular hyaluronidase; e.g. hylase) or ovine origin (ovine testicular hyaluronidase; e.g. vitrase.

The physiological role of hyaluronidase is seen in stimulating angiogenesis by defragmenting HA and in the fibrotic healing of adult and late gestational wounds.[53]

Hyaluronidase acts as a regulatory agent in HA homeostasis and metabolism.[54] Hyaluronidase cannot cross the blood-brain barrier.[55]

❑ PRACTICAL CONSIDERATION

Although there are no large randomized controlled trials on the efficacy of hyaluronidase in reducing unwanted depots of HA, it is a life saver in an injectors practice especially those who have a higher usage of HA fillers. Based on the reviewed literature some practical considerations can be given.

In the case of unwanted depots of HA, the following steps should be performed:

- Inform the patient that in rare cases, adverse reactions to the hyaluronidase have been known. Do not skin test. The allergic reactions are quite rare and cannot totally be excluded by skin test (Figure 24)
- Do not treat patients with a known allergy to bovine protein if the hyaluronidase used derives from bovine material
- There are many ways to diluting; which is specific to the type of hyaluronidse. However, the most common one used and available in India is hylase and it can be diluted by mixing the hyaluronidase (150 U vial) with 0.9% saline 1 mL) and injecting the mixture in the HA depots. There is no evidence that the addition of lidocaine or epinephrine is helpful. The volume used depends on the quantity of injected HA. Usually 0.05–0.1 mL per injection point (7.5–15 U) is sufficient. Inject slowly
- Choose the needle size according to the location and the size of the depot. Use a 30 G (0.3–13 mm) needle for more superficial nodules and a 27 G (0.4–20 mm), or a 26 G (0.45–10 mm) needle for deeper nodules
- Make sure to inject in the HA depot; in cases of very superficial HA depots, inject just beneath the depot
- For nodules exclusively due to HA, some patients notice an obvious decrease or a disappearance of the nodule within 24–

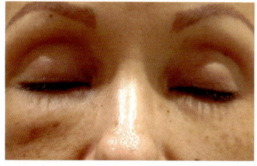
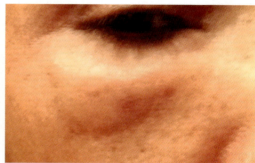

Figure 24: Hypersensitivity to hyaluronidase.

48 hours. For nodules of unknown cause, an obvious reduction of inflammation and size has been induced in some patients. Usually, an apparent regression is noticeable within 24–48 hours; however, in inflamed nodules a complete disappearance may take longer. Therefore, a follow-up visit should be scheduled about 2 weeks after the injection

- If the nodule is very inflamed and an abscess may be likely, an adjuvant systemic antibiotic treatment, e.g. with ciprofloxacine (500 mg twice a day) or levofloxacine 500 mg once daily, should be initiated as hyaluronidase may act as the spreading factor. Therefore, it is best to cover with antibiotics and wait for a few days after which hyaluronidase can be injected.

❏ CONCLUSION

The past decade has seen the arrival of a host of new soft tissue fillers for facial rejuvenation, which not only smoothen wrinkles but also have the ability to restore facial volume to create a balanced, more natural look.

A "complication free" procedure becomes an enjoyable experience for both the patient and the injector and to achieve this, the practicing physician should be suitably experienced to select different filler products accordingly to their properties, which will necessitate a detailed understanding of the facial anatomy, proper preparation and injection techniques and correct placement of the product.

Most adverse events are avoidable with proper planning and technique. As an injector matures and masters his craft, one of the most gratifying aspects is patient retention over the decades. Superior aesthetic results which can be almost risk free is a possibility and every injector must endeavor to achieve this in their injectable practice.

❏ REFERENCES

1. Goldberg DJ. Legal ramifications of off-label filler use. Dermatol Ther. 2006;19(3):189-93.
2. Rzany B, Hilton S, Prager W, et al. Expert guideline on the use of porcine collagen in aesthetic medicine. J Dtsch Dermatol Ges. 2010;8(3):210-7.
3. Rohrich RJ, Pessa JE. The retaining system of the face: Histologic evaluation of the septal boundaries of the subcutaneous fat compartments. Plast Reconstr Surg. 2008;121:1804-9.
4. Rohrich RJ, Pessa JE. The fat compartments of the face: Anatomy and clinical implications for cosmetic surgery. Plast Reconstr Surg. 2007;119:2219-31. discussion 2228-31.
5. Donofrio LM. Fat distribution: A morphologic study of the aging face. Dermatol Surg. 2000;26:1107-12.
6. American Society for Aesthetic Plastic Surgery Cosmetic surgery national data bank statistics 2012. Available from: http://www.surgery.org/sites/default/fles/ASAPS-2011-Stats.pdf. [Accessed September 13, 2013].
7. Zielke H, Wölber L, Wiest L, Rzany B. Risk profiles of different injectable fillers: results from the Injectable Filler Safety Study (IFS Study). Dermatol Surg. 2008;34(3):326-35.
8. Funt D, Pavicic T. Dermal fillers in aesthetics: an overview of adverse events and treatment approaches. Clin Cosmet Investig Dermatol. 2013;6:295-316.
9. Cohen JL, Bhatia AC. The role of topical vitamin K oxide gel in the resolution of postprocedural purpura. J Drugs Dermatol. 2009;8:1020-4.
10. Van Dyke S, Hays GP, Caglia AE, Caglia M. Severe Acute Local Reactions to a Hyaluronic Acid-derived Dermal Filler. J Clin Aesthet Dermatol. 2010;3(5):32-5.
11. Funt D, Pavicic T. Dermal fillers in aesthetics: an overview of adverse events and treatment. Clin Cosmet Investig Dermatol. 2013;6:295-316.
12. Geisler D, Shumer S, Elson ML. Delayed hypersensitivity reaction to Restylane®. Cosmetic Dermatol. 2007;20(12):784-6.
13. Arron ST, Neuhaus IM. Persistent delayed-type hypersensitivity reaction to injectable non-animal-stabilized hyaluronic acid. J Cosmet Dermatol. 2007;6(3):167-71.
14. Cassuto D, Marangoni O, De Santis G, Christensen L. Advanced laser techniques for filler-induced complications. Dermatol Surg. 2009;35(Suppl 2):1689-95.
15. Pessa JE, Garza JR. The malar septum: the anatomic basis of malar mounds and malar edema. Aesthet Surg J. 1997;17(1):11-7.
16. Funt DK. Avoiding malar edema during midface/cheek augmentation with dermal fillers. J Clin Aesthet Dermatol. 2011;4(12):32-6.
17. Gladstone HB, Cohen JL. Adverse effects when injecting facial fillers. Semin Cutan Med Surg. 2007;26(1):34-9.

18. Hirsch RJ, Narurkar V, Carruthers J. Management of injected hyaluronic acid induced Tyndall effects. Lasers Surg Med. 2006;38(3):202-4.

19. Douse-Dean T, Jacob CI. Fast and easy treatment for reduction of the Tyndall effect secondary to cosmetic use of hyaluronic acid. J Drugs Dermatol. 2008;7(3):281-3.

20. Lemperle G, Rullan PP, Gauthier-Hazan N. Avoiding and treating dermal filler complications. Plast Reconstr Surg. 2006;118:92s-107s.

21. Lemperle G, Duffy DM. Treatment options for dermal filler complications. Aesthet Surg J. 2006;26:356-64.

22. Alam M, Gladstone H, Kramer EM, Murphy JP Jr, Nouri K, Neuhaus IM, et al. ASDS guidelines of care: injectable fillers. Dermatol Surg. 2008;34:S115-48.

23. Cohen JL. Understanding, avoiding, and managing dermal filler complications. Dermatol Surg. 2008;34:S92-9.

24. Graivier MH, Bass LS, Busso M, Jasin ME, Narins RS, Tzikas TL. Calcium hydroxylapatite (Radiesse) for correction of the mid- and lower face: consensus recommendations. Plast Reconstr Surg. 2007;120:55s-66s.

25. Beer KR. Radiesse nodule of the lips from a distant injection site: report of a case and consideration of etiology and management. J Drugs Dermatol. 2007;6:846-7.

26. Berlin A, Cohen JL, Goldberg DJ. Calcium hydroxylapatite for facial rejuvenation. Semin Cutan Med Surg. 2006;25:132-7.

27. Alam M, Dover JS. Management of complications and sequelae with temporary injectable fillers. Plast Reconstr Surg. 2007;120:98s-105s.

28. Jones D. Volumizing the face with soft tissue fillers. Clin Plast Surg. 2011;38:379-90.

29. Peter S, Mennel S. Retinal branch artery occlusion following injection of hyaluronic acid (Restylane). Clin Experiment Ophthalmol. 2006;34(4):363-4.

30. Kim YJ, Kim SS, Song WK, Lee SY, Yoon JS. Ocular ischemia with hypotony after injection of hyaluronic acid gel. Ophthal Plast Reconstr Surg. 2011;27(6):e152-5.

31. Kwon SG, Hong JW, Roh TS, Kim YS, Rah DK, Kim SS. Ischemic oculomotor nerve palsy and skin necrosis caused by vascular embolization after hyaluronic Acid filler injection: a case report. Ann Plast Surg. 2013;71(4):333-4.

32. Lee DH, Yang HN, Kim JC, Shyn KH. Sudden unilateral visual loss and brain infarction after autologous fat injection into nasolabial groove. Br J Ophthalmol. 1996;80(11):1026-7.

33. Silva MT, Curi AL. Blindness and total ophthalmoplegia after aesthetic polymethylmethacrylate injection: case report. Arq Neuropsiquiatr. 2004;62(3B):873-4.

34. De Boulle K. Management of complications after implantation of fillers. J Cosmet Dermatol. 2004;3:2-15.

35. Sclafani AP, Fagien S. Treatment of injectable soft tissue filler complications. Dermatol Surg. 2009;35:1672-80.

36. Kim SG, Kim YJ, Lee SI, Lee CJ. Salvage of nasal skin in a case of venous compromise after hyaluronic acid filler injection using prostaglandin E. Dermatol Surg. 2011;37:1817-9.

37. Dayan SH, Arkins JP, Mathison CC. Management of impending necrosis associated with soft tissue filler injections. J Drugs Dermatol. 2011;10:1007-12.

38. Sung HM, Suh IS, Lee HB, Tak KS, Moon KM, Jung MS. Case reports of adipose-derived stem cell therapy for nasal skin necrosis after filler injection. Arch Plast Surg. 2012;39:51-4.

39. Rongioletti F. Exogenous cutaneous deposits with special consideration to skin reactions to soft tissue fillers. In: Rongioletti F, Smoller BR, editors. Clinical and pathological aspects of skin diseases in endocrine, metabolic, nutritional and deposition disease. New York: Springer; 2010. p. 139-52.

40. Lemperle G, Gauthier-Hazan N. Foreign body granulomas after all injectable dermal fillers: part 2. Treatment options. Plast Reconstr Surg. 2009;123:1864-73.

41. Omranifard M, Taheri S. Filler augmentation, safe or unsafe: a case series of severe complications of fillers. J Res Med Sci. 2011;16:(12) 627-31.

42. Rongioletti F, Atzori L, Ferreli C, Pau M, Pinna AL, Mercuri SR, et al. Granulomatous reactions after multiple aesthetic micro-implants in temporal combinations: a complication of filler addiction. J Eur Acad Dermatol Venereol. 2015;29:1188-93.

43. Dadzie OE, Mahalingam M, Parada M, El Helou T, Philips T, Bhawan J. Adverse cutaneous reactions to soft tissue fillers—a review of the histological features.J Cutan Pathol. 2008;35:536-48.

44. Requena L, Requena C, Christensen L, Zimmermann US, Kutzner H, Cerroni L. Adverse reactions to injectable soft tissue fillers. J Am Acad Dermatol. 2011;64:1-34

45. Christensen L, Breiting V, Janssen M, Zimmermann US, Kutzner H, Cerroni L. Adverse reactions to injectable soft tissue permanent fillers. Aesthetic Plast Surg. 2005;29:34-48.

46. Requena C, Izquierdo MJ, Navarro M, Martínez A, Vilata JJ, Botella R, et al. Adverse reactions to injectable aesthetic microimplants. Am J Dermatopathol. 2001;23:197-202.

47. Vargas-Machuca I, Gonzalez-Guerra E, Angulo J, del Carmen Fariña M, Martín L, Requena L. Facial granulomassecondary to Dermalive microimplants: report of a case with histopathologic differential diagnosis among the granulomas secondary to different injectable permanent filler materials. Am J Dermatopathol. 2006;28:173-7.

48. Pecharki D, Petersen FC, Scheie AA. Role of hyaluronidase in Streptococcus intermedius biofilm. Microbiology. 2008; 154:932-8.

49. DeLorenzi C. Complications of injectable fillers, part I. Aesthet Surg J. 2013;33:561-75.

50. Bjarnsholt T, Tolker-Nielsen T, Givskov M, Janssen M, Christensen LH. Detection of bacteria by fluorescence in situ hybridization in culture-negative soft tissue filler lesions. Dermatol Surg. 2009;35(Suppl 2):1620-4.

51. Cavallini M, Antonioli B, Gazzola R, Tosca M, Galuzzi M Rapisarda V, et al. Hyaluronidases for treating complications by hyaluronic acid dermal fillers: evaluation of the effects on cell cultures and human skin. Eur J Plast Surg. 2013;36(8):477-84.

52. Lee A, Grummer SE, Kriegel D, Marmur E. Hyaluronidase. Dermatol Surg. 2010, 36:1071-7

53. West DC, Shaw DM, Lorenz P, Adzick NS, Longaker MT. Fibrotic healing of adult and late gestation fetal wound correlates with increased hyaluronidase activity and removal of hyaluronan. Int J Biochem Cell Biol. 1997;9(1):201-10.

54. Schwartz DM, Jumper MD, Lui GM, Dang S, Schuster S,Stern R. Corneal endothelial hyaluronidase: a role in anterior chamber hyaluronic acid catabolism. Cornea. 1997;16(2):188-91.

55. Jiang D, Liang J, Noble PW. Hyaluronan in tissue injury and repair. Annu Rev Cell Dev Biol. 2007;23:435-61.

Complications of Injectable Botulinum Toxin for Cosmetic Indications

Rajetha Damisetty

❏ INTRODUCTION

Botulinum exotoxin A injections for treatment of facial wrinkles is the most frequently performed cosmetic procedure in the United States. About 4.6 million cosmetic neurotoxin procedures were done in the year 2014 versus 67,000 in 1997, with a 5,400% increase in 17 years, compared to 0.6% increase in the number of chemical peels during the same period of time and a 51% increase in laser hair reduction procedures in the past 14 years.[1]

The low cost of investment, predictability of results, ease of administration, versatility of benefits, and short learning curve, especially when used in the upper half of the face, combined with the willingness of the urban cosmetic patient, make it an attractive procedure for both novice and established cosmetic dermatologists to incorporate into their practice.[2]

Botulinum toxin injections are generally considered safe in trained hands and no long term or debilitating adverse events have been reported when used for cosmetic indications.[3]

A review of 1,437 adverse event reports over 13.5 years (December 1989 to May 2003) and nonserious adverse events reported from December 2001 to November 2002 to the Food and Drug Administration (FDA) through the MedWatch system was published;[4] 406 followed therapeutic use of β-adrenergic agonist (BTA; 217 serious and 189 nonserious) and 1,031 followed cosmetic use (36 serious and 995 nonserious). Reported adverse events occurred predominantly in female patients, with a median age of 50 years. In the year December 2001 to November 2002, when both serious and nonserious reports were evaluated, the proportion of reports classified as serious was 33-fold higher for therapeutic than for cosmetic cases. The 217 serious adverse events reported in therapeutic cases involved a wide spectrum of events and included all 28 reported deaths. Among cosmetic users, no deaths were reported and, of the 36 serious adverse events, 30 were included as possible complications in the FDA-approved label. The remaining 6 serious adverse events were deemed coincidental, with no causal relationship to BTA. About a third (13 of 36) of the patients with cosmetic use and serious adverse events had an underlying disease that may have been related to the reported adverse event (e.g. a BTA user with asthma was reported with respiratory compromise after BTA injection; a BTA user with a history of heart murmur was reported with arrhythmia post-BTA injection).

Among the 995 cosmetic cases reported to have nonserious adverse events, most commonly noted were lack of effect (623, 63%), injection site reaction (190, 19%), and ptosis (111, 11%).

Adverse events due to botulinum toxin may be classified as:

- Serious adverse events
- Immune mediated events, which may or may not be serious
- Nonserious adverse events.

❑ SERIOUS ADVERSE EVENTS

The lethal dose of botulinum toxin type A is between 2,500 and 3,000 units (U) for a 70 kg person, which is much higher than the typical dosage used for cosmetic applications (usually below 100 U).[5] There are case reports of botulism with injected botulinum toxin; however, these instances involved research-grade botulinum toxin that was not approved or intended for human use.[6,7]

Adverse events were classified as serious[4] if they met the United States Code of Federal Regulations 600.80 regulatory definition: "...death, a life-threatening adverse drug experience, in-patient hospitalization or prolongation of existing hospitalization, a persistent or significant disability/incapacity, or a congenital anomaly/birth defect... or ...intervention to prevent one of [these outcomes]..."

Respiratory compromise, flu-like syndrome, cardiac arrhythmias, precipitation of myasthenia gravis, focal muscle weakness, seizures, dysphagia, ptosis, retinal detachment/vitreous detachment/optic nerve atrophy, severe vomiting, malaise, and intractable headache have been reported in a small number of patients in the 30 serious adverse events attributed to the toxin.[4] Pseudoaneurysm of the superficial temporal artery following neurotoxin injection is also considered a serious adverse event.

Temporal Artery Pseudoaneurysm

There are two documented cases of superficial temporal artery pseudoaneurysm related to cosmetic botulinum toxin injection.[8,9] In the first case report, 30 U of botulinum toxin were injected (the report does not specify the distribution), and the patient presented 6 months later with a 2 cm by 4 cm pulseless forehead mass. The second patient was injected with 4 U botulinum toxin A above the eyebrows and 6 U within the left lateral periorbital area, and presented 2 months later with a nontender, nonmobile, nonerythematous pulsating mass. Immediately after the procedures, there was bruising over the area where the pseudoaneurysm would develop. Both pseudoaneurysms were confirmed by Doppler ultrasound. The first patient was treated surgically; the second was successfully treated without recurrence via intra-arterial embolization.

A pseudoaneurysm forms after direct vessel trauma, with resultant hematoma and capsule formation. As the hematoma resorbs and the capsule remains, the result is a cavity that communicates with the injured vessel.[8] The mechanism of injury in the case of botulinum injection-related temporal artery pseudoaneurysm formation is most likely direct penetration of the needle into the vessel.[8] The anterior branch of the superficial temporal artery is the most vulnerable to injury because of its location in the lateral forehead. As the vessel passes over the frontal osseous ridge, it is invested and tethered by the fascia of the temporalis muscle, which prevents the artery from being pushed aside during injection. Diagnosis is suggested by a pulsatile mass seen in the characteristic anatomic location over the lateral forehead. Fremitus and bruit may be heard on physical exam, and compression of the proximal artery may abolish or decrease these findings. Diagnosis is established by Doppler ultrasound, computed tomography, or angiography, which are the gold standards. Therapeutic options include surgical resection, ligation, sclerosis, ultrasound-guided thrombin injection, and coil embolization.[8]

Immune Mediated Reactions

Toxemia-like reactions including nausea, malaise, flu-like symptoms, and cutaneous eruptions may result from diffusion of neurotoxin into the systemic circulation, and are treated symptomatically. Systemic reactions are considered hypersensitivity to botulinum toxin or one of the components (i.e. albumin or lactose) in the suspension.[4] Allergies are rare, but case reports of fixed drug eruption,[10] localized anaphylactic reaction of the leg,[11] and development of sarcoidal nodules from antigenic stimulation following injection[12] have been reported. One fatal case of anaphylaxis was reported from a Botox-lidocaine mixture for therapeutic uses;[13] however, there are no reports of anaphylaxis for cosmetic purposes.

❑ NONSERIOUS ADVERSE EVENTS

Nonserious adverse events caused by botulinum toxin may be classified as:
- Nonresponse or failure to meet expectations of the patient
- Local events due to the injection per se
- Unaesthetic effects due to dosage maladjustment or improper placement of injections
- Distant ones due to inadvertent diffusion of the toxin.

Nonresponse to Botulinum Toxin

The most common reason for nonresponse is loss of potency of the protein due to freezing of the reconstituted product, break in the cold chain without storing the product between 4–8 degrees centigrade and using the solution way beyond the recommended period of 4 weeks after reconstitution.[14]

Prevalence of neutralizing antibodies is reported to be less than 5%. This may lead to secondary nonresponse. An estimated 5–15% of patients injected serially with 79–11 Botox (available in the early part of 21st century) developed secondary nonresponsiveness from the production of neutralizing antibodies. Risk factors associated with the development of neutralizing antibodies include injection of more than 200 U per session and repeat or booster injections given within 1 month of treatment.[15] The BCB 2024 Botox available since late 1990s appears to have a lower potential to induce antibody production because of its decreased protein load.[16] When a patient loses his or her response, serum can be tested for neutralizing antibodies, although this rarely is performed outside research settings.

When secondary nonresponse is encountered due to presence of antibodies, botulinum toxin type B may be tried. However, it has to be noted that type B exotoxin is not approved for cosmetic indications by the FDA. No information is available as to whether neutralizing antibodies resolve over time and, consequently, whether attempts at reinjection should be made after a prolonged period.

In all patients with nonresponse, repeat injection with freshly reconstituted neurotoxin from a carefully handled vial should be done, to rule out loss of potency of the toxin due to breach in the cold chain. Using the lowest dose of toxin necessary to achieve the desired clinical effect and avoiding reinjection within 1 month appears prudent in an effort to keep antibody formation as low and unlikely as possible.[15]

Failure to Meet Expectations of the Patient

This can be avoided by choosing patients prudently and aligning expectations before the procedure, especially when deep static lines exist. Patients should be aligned that static lines can only be softened and even a filler or resurfacing with ablative or nonablative fractional lasers done in combination with the injectable neurotoxin might not efface the deep wrinkles completely. It is important to decide the dosage depending on whether the patient wants complete relaxation of the muscle or a mere softening of the dynamic lines.[2]

Patients with body dysmorphic disorder[17] should not be treated with the injectable to avoid litigation and bad-mouthing. It is best to deny or defer treatment for patients with unrealistic goals and expectations, fears of treatment, or an unstable psychologic status.[18]

Incomplete muscle paralysis with residual rhytides can be tackled by doing a "touch-up" after 2 weeks of initial treatment.[19]

Local Adverse Events

Pain, edema, erythema, and ecchymosis are the most commonly reported side effects of injectable neurotoxin.[18] Side effects of topical anesthesia used to make the toxin injection more comfortable may also be encountered.[20]

Pain

Injection site pain can be reduced by topical anesthesia using eutectic mixture of local anesthetics (EMLA; prilocaine and lidocaine 2.5% each) cream[21] or the more potent mixture of tetracaine and lidocaine 7.5% each, under occlusion for around an hour. However, edema and erythema due to the cream may occur, especially with the latter preparation. Small gauge needles (30–32 G),[22] using each needle for no more than 4–5 pricks, insertion of the needle through the pilosebaceous unit and pinching the skin before injection may reduce pain too.[23] Using the "gate theory" of pain and "tapping" an area near the injection site with the non-dominant hand of the injector or cooling the skin[24] before and after injection would confuse the neurons into feeling the vibration/temperature change rather than the pain of injection.

It is important to reconstitute the freeze-dried toxin powder using saline as severe pain can ensue when distilled water is used. It is best to reconstitute with preserved saline instead of nonpreserved saline as pain can be reduced further without changing efficacy or safety.[24]

Pain is relatively less when each needle is used for no more than 4–5 pricks as needles get blunt after multiple pricks and consequently induce more pain (author's experience and anecdotal reports).

Headaches were the most frequently reported adverse event in the initial trials of onabotulinum toxin for the treatment of glabellar lines (onabotulinum toxin, 15.3% and 11% vs. placebo, 15.0% and 20%), which is most likely a result of the injection technique and not the drug itself.[25] A case report of five patients receiving botulinum neurotoxin treatment for cosmetic purposes described severe and debilitating headaches that resolved with appropriate therapy and were postulated to occur from either the microtrauma of needle penetration into the periosteum or toxin-induced muscle spasm.[26] They remitted either spontaneously or with the aid of analgesics within days to weeks. Fortunately, headaches are usually mild and require no specific treatment.

Apprehension and pain, real or anticipated, related to the treatment may even lead to vasovagal syncope.[19]

Bruising

Injection site ecchymosis reportedly occurs in less than 1% of all injections and can be reduced by avoidance of nonessential anticoagulants such as aspirin, nonsteroidal anti-inflammatory drugs, herbal remedies (vitamin E, ginseng, ginger, ginkgo, garlic, kava-kava, celery root, fish oils, St. John's wort), smoking, and alcohol for 7–10 days before the procedure.[20] Patients with bleeding disorders and those on anticoagulant drugs should be treated with caution but are not required to stop their necessary treatments.[17] Such patients should be warned of the potential for extensive and prolonged bruising.

Superficial injection, after visualizing small vessels, and carefully avoiding them, should reduce bruising. Cold compresses and direct firm pressure immediately after injection can also mitigate the risk of postinjection bruising. Even with the use of proper technique and careful patient selection, the periocular, perioral, and lid margins, composed of thin skin with superficial vessels, are very prone to ecchymosis. Up to 25% of patients have demonstrated bruising after receiving treatment of the crow's feet (periocular) with onabotulinum toxin. Similar rates occurred in the placebo group, implying that the ecchymosis resulted from the injection rather than the toxin itself.[27]

Those patients who desire a form of prevention for bruising can be treated preoperatively with herbal remedies such as *Arnica montana* and/or bromelain, which have been shown to reduce bruising and swelling by both small clinical trials and anecdotally.[28,29] Topical *Arnica* was found to accelerate the resolution of laser induced bruising and may, purportedly, be useful in botulinum toxin injection induced bruising too.[30]

Opaque makeup is useful to conceal discoloration, and several excellent products are available commercially (Dermacolor, Dermablend Professional). Treatment with 595 nm pulsed dye laser can hasten resolution of ecchymoses by several days, with high patient satisfaction.[31]

Reactions to Topical Anesthesia

Erythema and edema consequent to application of EMLA (2.5% lidocaine and prilocaine each) may occur in a few patients. They are even more pronounced when mixture of tetracaine and lidocaine 7% each is used.[32] Allergic contact dermatitis to the constituents are probably responsible for this effect. Because allergic contact dermatitis is a delayed type IV hypersensitivity reaction (localized dermatitis), the risk of anaphylaxis is not a concern.[33] Both combinations are safe and well tolerated by most patients.

Unaesthetic Effects Due to Dosage Maladjustment or Improper Placement of Injections

Asymmetry

Asymmetry may occur due to dosage maladjustment, mainly because the size of the target muscle may not be equal; differential dosing may be required if the activity of the muscles is not equal on both sides of the face.

It is important to align the patient about pre-existing asymmetry and inform him/her that while an attempt to correct the asymmetry will be made by the injector, perfect symmetry might be achievable. Baseline photographs should be saved for corroboration. Complaint of asymmetry is common with the eyebrows.

Quizzical Eyebrow

Creation of a quizzical eyebrow (spocking, aka Mr Spock of Star trek, Figure 1) may happen when frontalis fibers over the lateral brow are not treated or undertreated. The lateral portion of the muscle, when left untreated, will continue to elevate the brow when contracted, with the medial frontalis paralyzed, only the lateral brow will elevate.

This can produce a dramatic change in eyebrow shape often referred to by patients as the "Jack Nicholson look", referring to a similarity with the eyebrow shape of the well-known Hollywood actor (Figure 2). Toxin

injection of 1–2 U high on the lateral forehead 3–4 cm above the brow at the point of lateral-most frontalis muscle activity (assessed by having the patient contract the muscle) would correct this hitch (Figure 3).[20]

Incidence of accidental lateral brow elevation from overzealous eyebrow depressors and/or mid-frontalis treatment cannot be estimated as this is easily corrected and reporting is not common.

Rippled Forehead

The upper frontalis fibers, near the hairline, when inadequately treated with botulium toxin, give a "rippled" appearance during movement. Both Spock's eyebrow and rippled upper frontalis are obvious clinical signs the patient has been treated with neurotoxin.[23]

Exacerbation of Lower Eyelid "Bags"

Infraorbital crow's feet are treated with an injection into this part of the orbicularis

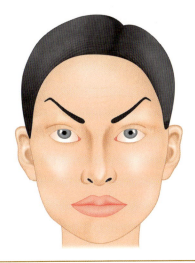

Figure 1: Mr Spock-like eyebrows.

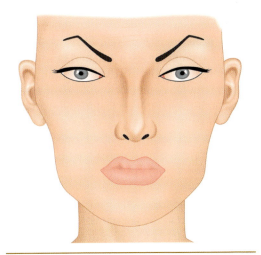

Figure 2: Quizzical eyebrows.

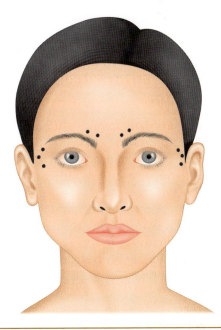

Figure 3: Points of injection for correction of quizzical eyebrows.

oculi 5–6 mm below the lash margin, in the midpupillary line. Midpupillary line injections of the lower eyelid should only be performed in patients with a positive snap test (good lower lid elasticity). In older patients with poor skin recoil, sagginess of the lower lid increases when the underlying muscle is relaxed.

A dose finding study[34] found doses greater than 4 U in the lower eyelid were associated with complications such as an inability to completely close the eye and photophobia. Some patients may experience infraorbital puffiness at even smaller doses and all should be warned of this possibility prior to treatment.

Mask-like Face/Frozen Forehead

Many patients are apprehensive of this consequence of neurotoxin injection as it is a tell-tale sign of treatment and most patients with purely cosmetic concerns desire a natural look and are not comfortable confession that they underwent aesthetic procedures. Keeping injections 3 cm above the brow will lessen the risk of diminished expressiveness.[23]

❑ ADVERSE EVENTS DUE TO INADVERTENT DIFFUSION OF THE TOXIN

Local spread of botulinum toxin occurs by diffusion of up to 3 cm in diameter from the injection point.[5] Injection technique, injection volumes, concentration gradients, and anatomic boundaries influence local diffusion. Dilution volumes range from 1 to 4 mL per 100 U vial.[2] Most injectors use a dilution of 2.5 mL per 100 U, amounting to 4 U per 0.1 mL of solution and each unit corresponding to one marking in an insulin syringe with 40 markings per millimeter.

The concentration of neurotoxin is greatest at the point of injection, and the gradient decreases rapidly with distance from this point. Higher the concentration of toxin, lower the distance to which diffusion occurs. Hence, lower concentrations which necessitate higher volumes per site are more fraught with the risk of unintended diffusion and accidental muscle paralysis. In certain situations, it is helpful to consider lower dilutions that give higher localized concentrations and lower injection volumes to help reduce spread or unwanted diffusion. Most cosmetic physicians tell patients to stay upright for at least 3–4 hours after the procedure and avoid massaging the injected areas as a precautionary measure, despite lack of evidence to validate this routine in preventing unwanted effects.[23] They are also advised to avoid massaging or applying heat to the treatment area, and to avoid activities that cause flushing (such as exercising heavily, consuming alcohol, and hot tub use) on the day of treatment.[19] These aftercare practices are used to reduce potential spread of the toxin; however, they are not supported by randomized controlled trials.

Upper face botulinum toxin injections are generally far safer compared to lower face treatments, as interlacing of fibers of the numerous small muscles in the lower face increase the chances of unintended paralysis of adjacent muscles. Depth and site of injection have to be decided with utmost care; it is best to gain sufficient experience in basic upper face treatments of forehead horizontal lines, glabellar complex, crow's feet, and Bunny lines before venturing on to advanced indications such as brow lift, depressor anguli oris, mentalis, masseter injections, Nefertiti lift, and platysmal bands. Smaller doses fare used or perioral treatment than for upper facial applications as the oral musculature responds more strongly to the same botulinum toxin dosing.

Pre-existing anatomic asymmetries from genetics or previous surgery or trauma should be pointed out to the patient before treatment, and injection technique and dosing should be modified.

Brow ptosis, diplopia, lid ptosis, distorted smile, upper lip ptosis, neck weakness, dysphagia, and dry eye syndrome may occur as a consequence of inadvertent diffusion of the neurotoxin.

Brow Ptosis

Midbrow ptosis is probably more common and underreported in trials and clinical practice.[23] Lateral eyebrow ptosis has been reported in 5% of 183 patients undergoing treatment for periocular lines (crow's feet) in an early dose finding study with onabotulinum toxin (Botox).[35]

Treating horizontal forehead lines 2 weeks after glabellar frown lines may reduce occurrence of brow ptosis in first-time patients. Isolated frontalis treatments should be avoided, as unopposed brow depressor action of procerus and corrugators may lead to brow ptosis.

It is best to test for occult/compensated brow or lid ptosis prior to treatment. Compensated ptosis is noted when patients raise the eyebrow to compensate for a ptotic or drooping eyelid, and can be tested for by relaxing the brow and assessing lid position. Injections should be kept at least 1 cm above the orbital rim to avoid ptosis.

In case frontalis alone is treated, treating brow depressors (glabellar complex, lateral brow) may counteract mild brow ptosis. Alpha-adrenergic agonist eye drops stimulate Müller's muscle to counteract a weakened eyelid levator muscle and help disguise eyelid and mild brow ptosis.

Overtreatment of the inferior forehead can result in eyebrow depression and inability to elevate the brow, with a resultant sad, heavy appearance. Care should be taken not to overtreat the forehead and to remember that the lower 2 cm of the frontalis is responsible for brow position (Figures 4 and 5).

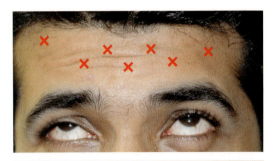

Figure 4: Points of injection for frontalis, avoiding the lower 2 cm to maintain brow position and prevent frozen forehead.

Source: Derma-Care, Mangaluru.

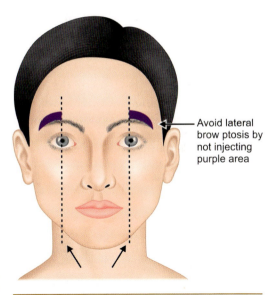

Avoid lateral brow ptosis by not injecting purple area

Figure 5: Avoiding danger zone, to prevent brow ptosis.

Strabismus and Diplopia

There are several published case series of strabismus and resultant diplopia following botulinum toxin treatment of lateral canthal rhytids.[36,37] Diplopia typically began 1–2 weeks following treatment. In 3 cases, the diplopia resolved without treatment over the course of 3 months.[37] Brazilian oculoplastic surgeons described two patients who developed diplopia after periocular cosmetic use of botulinum toxin A. They were treated with intramuscular botulinum toxin A injection into the antagonist extraocular muscle. Diplopia resolved in both patients in less than 1 week with no side effects or complications.[38]

The proposed mechanism for strabismus after periocular botulinum toxin injection was infiltration of the toxin due to diffusion into the orbit to the extraocular muscles with subsequent paralysis.[38] The risk is increase when technique is poor or large volumes are used.

Most cases were associated with lateral rectus paralysis; however, medial rectus paralysis was encountered with nasalis injections.

Staying at least 1 cm lateral to the orbital rim (>1.5 cm from the lateral canthus) will help to avoid diplopia, strabismus, and lid ptosis (Figure 6).

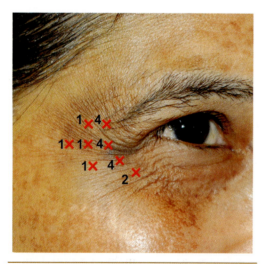

Figure 6: Points of injection for lateral crow's feet, avoiding the zygomatic muscles and maintaining 1 cm distance from orbital margin.

Source: Derma-Care, Mangaluru.

Blepharoptosis (Upper Eyelid Ptosis)

Blepharoptosis is caused by deep migration of botulinum toxin through the orbital septum fascia to the levator palpebrae superioris, an upper eyelid levator muscle. It is mostly encountered when corrugator supercilii muscles are injected to relax the frown. It may also happen when lateral brow lift is attempted by relaxing the orbicularis oculi.

Incidence of blepharoptosis is reduced by placing botulinum toxin injections at least 1 cm above the supraorbital ridge at the midpupillary line when treating the corrugator muscles.[23] Temporary blepharoptosis is uncommon (1–5%), but is distressing for patients. It is almost always unilateral, seen as a 2–3 mm lowering of the affected eyelid that is most marked at the end of the day with muscle fatigue. Botox package insert reports blepharoptosis occurred in 3% of 405 individuals, whereas a large multicenter study noted 5.4% of patients (11 of 203), with no cases reported in the placebo group for patients treated with glabellar lines.[39,40] Even smaller percentages are reported in the package insert of abobotulinum toxin (Dysport) (2% vs. placebo, 1%).[41]

Blepharoptosis may be treated using ophthalmic solutions that have α-adrenergic effects, such as naphazoline 0.025%, pheniramine 0.3%, or apraclonidine 0.5%. These medications cause contraction of Müller muscle, an adrenergic levator muscle of the upper eyelid, resulting in elevation of the upper eyelid. Apraclonidine is reserved for refractory cases and should be used with caution because it can exacerbate or unmask underlying glaucoma.[42]

Most injectors prefer to reassure the patient about the transient nature of the adverse event rather than use these medications which have too short-lived an action to make a significant difference.

To limit the incidence of unwanted paralysis of the sole eyelid elevator, the following precautions may be taken.

- Grasping the area before injection to localize delivery
- Injecting in a perpendicular or upward direction rather than downward toward the orbit and massaging the injection site upward when completed
- Placing corrugator injections at least 1 cm above the orbital rim, orbicularis oculi injections at least 1–2 cm from the lateral orbital rim, and placing frontalis muscle injections at least 2.5 cm above the upper line of the eyebrow.
- Injecting >1 cm lateral to the orbital rim (>1.5 cm from the lateral canthus) to avoid both diplopia and lid ptosis
- Applying digital pressure, with the noninjecting thumb, along the orbital rim between the injection sites and the eye may also reduce eyelid ptosis
- The right depth of injection also prevents inadvertent deep injections into levator palpebrae superioris
- Procerus—inject 3 bevel deep, using 30 G needle with insulin syringe
- Body of the corrugator—inject 2 bevel deep
- Lateral corrugators—inject 1 bevel deep superficially.

It is possible that in spite of the above mentioned precautions and utmost care, a small subset of patients develop eyelid ptosis after injection of corrugators or orbicularis oculi. These patients may have an anatomical variation of levator palpebrae superioris' fibers inserting more anteriorly and superficially than usual. They may be treated safely by using more concentrated solution of botulinum toxin to limit the diffusion distance.

Distorted Smile and Upper Lip Ptosis

When injecting into or around the lip, there is high potential for lip ptosis, as many muscles of facial expression are involved in the movement and shape of the lips. When injecting the mentalis, depressor anguli oris, or orbicularis oris, unwanted spread or unintentional injection into the depressor labii inferioris may result in difficulty depressing the lower lip, resulting in an abnormal/asymmetrical smile and/or difficulty when eating. Inadvertent treatment of the zygomaticus major when treating the lower orbicularis oculi and nasalis or over-treatment of the levator labii superioris alaeque nasi when treating "gummy smile" can also cause an abnormal smile, as these muscles control the movement and shape of the upper lip and lip corners. Zygomaticus major and minor muscles that have their origin on the upper cheek near the malar eminence. Toxin migration can affect these muscles and reduce the ability of the patient to elevate the corner of the mouth.

An extensive analysis of 485 patients treated for various cosmetic purposes with botulinum toxin type A reported that of 20 patients injected in the middle and lower face, only 2 patients experienced partial lip ptosis following injection into the upper lip for treatment of nasolabial folds.[43]

Additionally, partial lip ptosis occurred in 3 cases in over 1,000 patients following injection of 7.5 units of botulinum toxin A to the lateral canthal rhytides (crow's feet); however, these patients had all undergone previous blepharoplasties, suggesting that altered anatomical planes may have resulted in toxin diffusion.[44]

Care should be taken to keep mentalis injections low and central in the mentalis. If toxin is injected laterally, it can affect the depressor labii inferioris and produce lower lip weakening and an asymmetrical smile.

Relaxation of the depressor anguli oris is accomplished by injecting 2–6 U into the depressor anguli oris in its posterior edge. This point is chosen so as to decrease the chance of weakening the muscle more medial to depressor anguli oris, the depressor labii inferioris. The point of injection is at the mandibular angle 1 cm lateral to the corner of the mouth.

Treatment of nasolabial fold rhytides with botulinum toxin A injection is practiced at times. The intended targets of muscle paralysis are the levator labii superioris alaeque nasi, which act to move the nasolabial fold and upper lip medially. Care must be taken when treating this muscle as there is a high tendency to create a droop of the upper lip.

There is no treatment for this condition, and patients must be reassured that this effect is temporary.

Functional Deficit of the Lips

Neurotoxin treatment should be avoided treatment for the vermillion border, depressor angularis oris, and mentalis in patients whom lip impairment could affect quality of life, such as musicians.[23]

Injections into the depressor anguli oris muscle should be kept away (lateral) from the depressor labii inferioris muscle and the mouth to avoid an asymmetric smile and incompetent mouth, which may lead to drooling while drinking or eating.

Neck Weakness, Hoarseness, and Dysphagia

The senescent changes seen in the neck are primarily due to the downward pull of the platysmal muscle over time, creating jowls, loss of definition of the chin and jawline, vertical fibrous bands, and multiple horizontal rhytides. Cervical botulinum toxin injections are used to reverse or reduce these changes. Most patients are given approximately 50–100 U of botulinum toxin per session; some authors feel comfortable using up to 200 U per session, but others remark that this increases the risk for complications.[45]

Cervical complications include neck weakness, hoarseness, and dysphagia.[45] The mechanism by which botulinum toxin causes these complications is presumed to be either local diffusion or direct injection of the toxin into the sternocleidomastoid and the strap muscles, laryngeal muscles, or muscles of deglutition, respectively.[46] Like most other complications of botulinum toxin injections, the cervical complications are reversible. These risks can be reduced by using less than 100 U of neurotoxin per session when treating the neck, and meticulous care to not inject past the thin platysma muscle to deeper structures. If dysphagia is noted, the patient's diet should be transitioned to soft liquid diet. Metoclopramide might prove useful as a gastrointestinal motility agent to improve swallowing.[46]

Injecting bands that are sandwiched between the thumb and forefinger of the noninjecting hand with very superficial, low doses will reduce these adverse events.[46]

Dry Eye Syndrome

There are a number of published case reports of patients developing xerophthalmia after botulinum toxin treatment of lateral crow's feet.

There are two major proposed mechanisms:
- Direct diffusion of toxin into the lacrimal gland to decrease secretory function[47]
- Lagophthalmos secondary to paralysis of the orbicularis oculi causing decreased tone and blink strength.[48]

Dry eye syndrome may be categorized into a spectrum of disease severity. Mild disease may manifest as eye irritation, foreign body sensation, or subtle blink dysfunction. Moderate disease as red eye, exposure keratitis, lid edema, scleral show, or moderate epiphora. Severe disease presents as photophobia, ectropion, and corneal erosion.[49] By early recognition of mild symptoms, and discontinuing botulinum toxin treatment, the vast majority of complications will self-resolve in approximately 3–6 months. However, permanent paralysis of facial muscles has been observed in patients treated with the neurotoxin for 1.5–2 years and one group noted that approximately 1% of patients treated for over 1 year had persistent moderate symptoms.[50]

Snap-back and distraction tests be performed before any periocular botulinum toxin injection to test for poor tone and contractility of the orbicularis oculi muscles.[50] The snap-back test involves pulling the lower eyelid downward, while the patient looks straight ahead without blinking. The eyelid should "snap-back" soon after the traction is released and before the patient blinks. The distraction test involves pulling the lower eyelid away from the globe and measuring the distance between globe and central lid margin in millimeters.

By incorporating these tests and inquiring about early symptoms of dry eye, it is possible to detect patients at risk for serious ocular complications and discontinue, at least temporarily, botulinum toxin treatment. The risk of dry eye syndrome can also be reduced by cautiously avoiding the "orbital zone" (1 cm radius around the orbit). Dry eye symptoms can be managed conservatively with preservative free lubricant eye drops. Prompt consultation with an ophthalmologist should be considered if symptoms are persistent or more severe. For persistent complications of dry eye unresponsive to conservative treatment over a 1-year course, surgical management like lateral musculoplasty can be considered.[51]

Complications Unique to Masseter Injections

Masseter treatments with botulinum toxin are a very convenient way of sculpting and

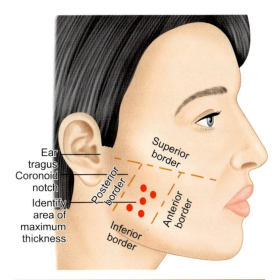

Figure 7: Points of botulinum toxin injection for masseter.

slimming the lower face, to convert a squarish broad jaw into a narrow oval feminine one. They have become popular, in spite of masseter injection being an off-label indication.

Temporary weakening of the ability to chew, minor changes in facial expression due to diffusion into zygomaticus major and buccinator may occur. Muscle may shrink faster than the overlying skin can contract, leading to temporary, usually subtle skin "sagging" postinjection. Patients may complain of relative prominence of temporalis and sunken cheek appearance, especially if zygoma is prominent. These can be avoided by following the guidelines[52] for identifying the muscle bulk (Figure 7) and using a long needle unlike the 6 or 8 mm 30 G needles usually used.

❑ CONTRAINDICATIONS TO BOTULINUM TOXIN USAGE

Certain medications that can interfere with neuromuscular transmission (i.e., amino-glycosides, muscle relaxants, or anticholinergic drugs), pregnancy and lactation, geriatric use (age >65 years), previous surgical alterations to the facial anatomy, marked facial asymmetry, inflammation or infection at the proposed injection site(s), ptosis, excessive dermatochalasis, deep dermal scarring, and hypersensitivity to any of the toxin preparation or components in the formulation. The contraindications are listed in table 1.

TABLE 1: Contraindications to botulinum toxin injection[19]
Body dysmorphic disorder
Unrealistic expectations
Dependency on facial expression for livelihood (e.g., actors, singers)
Dermatoses in the treatment area (e.g., psoriasis, eczema)
Gross motor weakness in the treatment area (e.g., Bell's palsy); botulinum toxin may be used to correct asymmetry by injecting the unaffected side
Immunocompromised
Infection in the treatment area
Keloidal scarring (traditionally described but frequently ignored, without any consequence)
Neuromuscular disorder (e.g., amyotrophic lateral sclerosis, myasthenia gravis, Lambert-Eaton syndrome, myopathies)
Pregnancy or breastfeeding
Sensitivity or allergy to constituents of the botulinum toxin product [e.g., cow's milk protein allergy with abobotulinum toxin A (Dysport)]

❑ LITIGATION

Lawsuits related to botulinum toxins are uncommon. A study of litigation between 1985 and 2012 found 24 relevant cases, all involving onabotulinumtoxinA. Lawsuits were 5 times more likely in therapeutic use of toxins with cases citing up to 600 U dosed. Allergan, Inc. was named in all cases; in only 3 cases were physicians named as codefendants. Only one case involved a dermatologist.[53]

❑ CONCLUSION

Botulinum toxin treatments for cosmetic injections are the most popular aesthetic treatments in the developed world and can be used safely and effectively, with enormous patient satisfaction.[2]

Botox (onabotulinumtoxinA) is the most commonly used botulinum toxin.[54] It appears to be less fragile and more stable than initially thought. While it is wise to follow the manufacturers' recommendations, some of them seem somewhat excessive. In cosmetic applications, botulinum toxin was initially used for treatment of upper facial dynamic rhytides, but is now considered a key component of facial rejuvenation procedures as an adjunct to either nonsurgical or surgical interventions, including in the lower face and neck.

Reduction of unwanted paralysis can be reduced through proper injection and dilution techniques. Application of pressure immediately postinjection, the use of lower dilutions with higher concentrations (lower injection volumes), placement of corrugator injections greater than 1 cm above the orbital bony rim, orbicularis oculi muscle injections at least 1–2 cm from the lateral orbital rim, and frontalis injections at least 2.5 cm above the mid-brow can all help limit unwanted diffusion.

Most complications are technique-dependent; incidence declines as injector skill improves.[49]

Botulinum toxin injectors should be well versed in diagnosing and managing complications. Counseling patients about the possibility of complications and taking a comprehensive informed consent would go a long way in protecting the injector during litigation.[53] Thorough knowledge of anatomy of facial musculature,[55] careful assessment and planning of injection dosage, sites, and depth in every patient would ensure reproducible, safe, and pleasing aesthetic results, along with garnering goodwill of the patient and likelihood of repeat treatments.

❏ REFERENCES

1. American Society for Aesthetic Plastic Surgery. Cosmetic Surgery National Data Bank statistics 2014. Available from: http://www.surgery.org/sites/default/files/2014-Stats.pdf. Accessed October 30, 2015.

2. Small R. Aesthetic procedures in office practice. Am Fam Physician. 2009;80(11):1231-7.

3. Naumann M, Jankovic J. Safety of botulinum toxin type A: a systematic review and meta-analysis. Curr Med Res Opin. 2004;20:981-90.

4. Coté TR, Mohan AK, Polder JA, Walton MK, Braun MM. Botulinum toxin type A injections: Adverse events reported to the US Food and Drug Administration in therapeutic and cosmetic cases. J Am Acad Dermatol. 2005;53:407-15.

5. Huang W, Foster JA, Rogachefsky AS. Pharmacology of botulinum toxin. J Am Acad Dermatol. 2000;43:249-59.

6. Souayah N, Karim H, Kamin SS, McArdle J, Marcus S. Severe botulism after focal injection of botulinum toxin. Neurology. 2006;67(10):1855-6.

7. Chertow DS, Tan ET, Maslanka SE, Schulte J, Bresnitz EA, Weisman RS, et al. Botulism in 4 adults following cosmetic injections with an unlicensed, highly concentrated botulinum preparation. JAMA. 2006;296(20):2476-9.

8. Prado A, Fuentes P, Guerra C, Leniz P, Wisnia P. Pseudoaneurysm of the frontal branch of the superficial temporal artery: an unusual complication after the injection of botox. Plast Reconstr Surg. 2007;119(7):2334-5.

9. Skaf GS, Domloj NT, Salameh JA, Atiyeh B. Pseudo-aneurysm of the superficial temporal artery: a complication of botulinum toxin injection. Aesthetic Plast Surg. 2012;36(4):982-5.

10. Cox NH, Duffey P, Royle J. Fixed drug eruption caused by lactose in an injected botulinum toxin preparation. J Am Acad Dermatol. 1999;40:263-4.

11. LeWitt PA, Trosch RM. Idiosyncratic adverse reactions to intramuscular botulinum toxin type A injection. Mov Disord. 1997;12:1064-7.

12. Ahbib S, Lachapelle JM, Marot L. Sarcoidal granulomas following injections of botulic toxin A (Botox) for corrections of wrinkles. Ann Dermatol Venereol. 2006;133:43-5.

13. Li M, Goldberger BA, Hopkins C. Fatal case of BOTOX-related anaphylaxis? J Forensic Sci. 2005;50:169-72.

14. Park MY, Ahn KY. Effect of the refrigerator storage time on the potency of botox for human extensor digitorum brevis muscle paralysis. J Clin Neurol. 2013;9(3):157-64.

15. Dressler D, Hallett M. Immunological aspects of botox, dysport and myobloc/neurobloc. Eur J Neurol. 2006;Suppl 1:11-5.

16. Jankovic J, Vuong KD, Ahsan J. Comparison of efficacy and immunogenicity of original versus current botulinum toxin in cervical dystonia. Neurology. 2003;60(7):1186-8.

17. Sommer B. How to avoid complications when treating hyperdynamic folds and wrinkles. Clin Dermatol. 2003;21(6):521-3.

18. Pena MA, Alam M, Yoo SS. Complications with the use of botulinum toxin type A for cosmetic applications and hyperhidrosis. Semin Cutan Med Surg. 2007;26:29-33.

19. Small R. Botulinum toxin injection for facial wrinkles. Am Fam Physician. 2014;90(3):168-75.

20. Levy LL, Emer JJ. Complications of minimally invasive cosmetic procedures: prevention and management. J Cutan Aesthet Surg. 2012;5(2):121-32.

21. Söylev MF, Koçak N, Kuvaki B, Ozkan SB, Kir E. Anesthesia with EMLA cream for botulinum A toxin injection into eyelids. Ophthalmologica. 2002;216:355–8.

22. Yomtoob DE, Dewan MA, Lee MS, Harrison AR. Comparison of pain scores with 30-gauge and 32-gauge needles for periocular botulinum toxin type a injections. Ophthal Plast Reconstr Surg. 2009; 25:376-7.

23. Emer J, Waldorf H. Injectable neurotoxins and fillers: there is no free lunch Clin Dermatol. 2011;29:678-90.

24. Linder JS, Edmonson BC, Laquis SJ, Drewry RD Jr, Fleming JC. Skin cooling before periocular botulinum toxin A injection. Ophthal Plast Reconstr Surg. 2002;18:441-2.

25. Carruthers JA, Lowe NJ, Menter MA, Gibson J, Nordquist M, Mordaunt J, et al. BOTOX Glabellar Lines I Study Group. A multicenter, double-blind, randomized, placebo-controlled study of the efficacy and safety of botulinum toxin type A in the treatment of glabellar lines. J Am Acad Dermatol. 2002;46:840-9.

26. Alam M, Arndt KA, Dover JS. Severe, intractable headache after injection with botulinum A exotoxin: report of 5 cases. J Am Acad Dermatol. 2002;46:62-5.

27. Lowe NJ, Lask G, Yamauchi P, Moore D. Bilateral, double-blind, randomized comparison of 3 doses of botulinum toxin type A and placebo in patients with crow's feet. J Am Acad Dermatol. 2002;47:834-40.

28. Broughton G 2nd, Crosby MA, Coleman J, Rohrich RJ. Use of herbal supplements and vitamins in plastic surgery: a practical review. Plast Reconstr Surg. 2007;119:48e-66e.

29. Kouzi SA, Nuzum DS. Arnica for bruising and swelling. Am J Health Syst Pharm. 2007;64:2434-43.

30. Leu S, Havey J, White LE, Martin N, Yoo SS, Rademaker AW, et al. Accelerated resolution of laser- induced bruising with topical 20% arnica: a rater-blinded randomized controlled trial. Br J Dermatol. 2010;163:557-63.

31. DeFatta RJ, Krishna S, Williams 3rd EF. Pulsed-dye laser for treating ecchymoses after facial cosmetic procedures. Arch Facial Plast Surg. 2009;11:99-103.

32. Cohen JL, Gold MH. Evaluation of the efficacy and safety of a lidocaine and tetracaine (7%/7%) cream for induction of local dermal anesthesia for facial soft tissue augmentation with hyaluronic Acid. J Clin Aesthet Dermatol. 2014;7(10):32-7.

33. To D, Kossintseva I, de Gannes G. Lidocaine contact allergy is becoming more prevalent. Dermatol Surg. 2014;40(12):1367-72.

34. Flynn TC, Carruthers JA, Carruthers JA, Clark RE 2nd. Botulinum A toxin (BOTOX) in the lower eyelid: dose finding study. Dermatol Surg. 2003;29:943-50.

35. Garcia A, Fulton JE Jr. Cosmetic denervation of the muscles of facial expression with botulinum toxin. A dose-response study. Dermatol Surg. 1996;2:39-43.

36. Sheen-Ophir S1, Almog Y. Diplopia following subcutaneous injections of botulinum toxin for cosmetic or medical use. Harefuah. 2013;152(2):98-100, 122-123.

37. Isaac CR, Chalita MR, Pinto LD. Botox® after Botox® - a new approach to treat diplopia secondary to cosmetic botulinic toxin use: case report. Arq Bras Oftalmol. 2012;75(3):213-4.

38. Ferreira MC, Salles AG, Gimenez R, Soares MF. Complications with the use of botulinum toxin type a in facial rejuvenation: Report of 8 cases. Aesthetic Plast Surg. 2004;28:441-4.

39. BOTOX cosmetic: package insert. Available from: http://www.allergan.com/assets/ pdf/botox_cosmetic_pi.pdf. Accessed December 15, 2010.

40. Carruthers JD, Lowe NJ, Menter MA, Gibson J, Eadie N; Botox Glabellar Lines II Study Group. Double-blind, placebo-controlled study of the safety and efficacy of botulinum toxin type A for patients with glabellar lines. Plast Reconstr Surg. 2003;112:1089-98.

41. Scottsdale AZ. Medicis Aesthetics Inc; 2009. Dysport.

42. Wollina U, Konrad H. Managing adverse events associated with botulinum toxin type A: a focus on cosmetic procedures. Am J Clin Dermatol. 2005;6(3):141-50.

43. Sarrabayrouse MA. Indications and limitations for the use of botulinum toxin for the treatment of facial wrinkles. Aesthetic Plast Surg. 2002;26:233-8.

44. Matarasso SL, Matarasso A. Treatment guidelines for botulinum toxin type A for the periocular region and a report on partial upper lip ptosis following injections to the lateral canthal rhytids. Plast Reconstr Surg. 2001;108:208-14. Discussion 215-7.

45. Matarasso A, Matarasso SL. Botulinum A exotoxin for the management of platysma bands. Plast Reconstr Surg. 2003;112(Suppl 5):s138-40.

46. Klein AW. Complications, adverse reactions, and insights with the use of botulinum toxin. Dermatol Surg. 2003;29(5):549-56.

47. Matarasso SL. Decreased tear expression with an abnormal Schirmer's test following botulinum toxin type A for the treatment of lateral canthal rhytides. Dermatol Surg. 2002;28(2):149-52.

48. Northington ME, Huang CC. Dry eyes and superficial punctate keratitis: a complication of treatment of glabelar dynamic rhytides with botulinum exotoxin A. Dermatol Surg. 2004;30(12 Pt 2):1515-7.

49. Sorensen EP, Urman C. Cosmetic complications: rare and serious events following botulinum toxin and soft tissue filler administration. J Drugs Dermatol. 2015;14(5):486-91.

50. Ozgur OK, Murariu D, Parsa AA, Parsa FD. Dry eye syndrome due to botulinum toxin type-A injection: guideline for prevention. Hawaii J Med Public Health. 2012;71(5):120-3.

51. Fogli AL. Orbicularis muscleplasty and face-lift: a better orbital contour. Plast Reconstr Surg. 1995;96(7):1560-70.

52. Liew S, Dart A. Nonsurgical reshaping of the lower face. Aesthetic Surg J. 2008;28:251-7.

53. Korman JB, Jalian HR, Avram MM. Analysis of botulinum toxin products and litigation in the United States. Dermatol Surg. 2013;39:1587-91.

54. Walker TJ, Dayan SH. Comparison and overview of currently available neurotoxins. J Clin Aesthet Dermatol. 2014;7(2):31-9.

55. Fagien S, Raspaldo H. Facial rejuvenation with botulinum neurotoxin: an anatomical and experimental perspective. J Cosmet Laser Ther. 2007;9(Suppl 1):23-31.

Complications of Mesotherapy

Amit Luthra

❏ INTRODUCTION

Mesotherapy (from Greek *mesos* meaning "middle" and therapy from Greek *therapeia*, "to treat medically") is a technique which involves microinjections of medications into the middle layer of the skin in order to improve musculoskeletal, neurologic and cosmetic conditions (Figure 1). In dermatology, it is used to target skin problems, such as dryness and dullness of the skin, cellulite and hair loss. Michel Pistor (1924–2003) performed clinical research and founded the field of mesotherapy. His concept was "A little, not so often and where you need it."

Multinational research in intradermal therapy culminated with Pistor's work from 1948 to 1952 in human mesotherapy treatments. The French press coined the term mesotherapy in 1958. The French Académie Nationale de Médecine recognized mesotherapy as a specialty of medicine in 1987.

It gained importance in France and gradually spread to other parts of Europe and America, especially when it was used to treat sport injuries. It has had its share of controversies with physicians against it, arguing on the lack of credible clinical and research evidence.

Following undesirable effects observed on several patients of a French practitioner, an official ratification was published in France in April 2011 to ban mesotherapy as a method for removing fat deposits. This ban was revoked in June 2011 by the French Council of State after investigation proved that these undesirable effects were not due to the painless injections of mesotherapy itself, but to the fact that it had been practiced in bad conditions and without respecting the hygiene principles.[1]

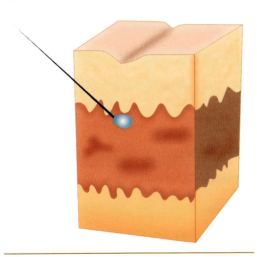

Figure 1: Level of mesotherapy injection.

❏ INDICATIONS AND TREATMENT METHODOLOGY

Most creams and topical skin treatments are limited by the poor penetration of the ingredients. Mesotherapy injections (shallow 1–4 mm injections) effectively deliver medication directly to areas that need it. These are almost spread evenly over a wide area.

Mesotherapy for all its criticisms, has some role in practice, especially cosmetic dermatology. It has been found to be useful for facial rejuvenation, cellulite reduction and hair loss treatment. Various terminologies (Flowchart 1) have been used like:

- Skin rejuvenation—mesoglow/mesolift
- Body sculpting—mesofat
- Hair growth—mesohair
- Stretch marks/loose skin—mesoboost.

Skin rejuvenation or facial rejuvenation has been divided into mesoglow, where vitamins are injected, mesoglow with hydration wherein vitamins are mixed with uncrosslinked hyaluronic acid and mesolift where uncrosslinked hyaluronic acid is injected intradermally in a point by point manner (by raising blebs) and even injected into lines and folds. Commercial preparations available in India for mesolift with hyaluronic acid are Restylane Vital, Mesolis, and IAL. Patients need to be selected keeping in mind the age of the patient and the condition of the skin (Table 1).

Protocols for the above mentioned would be as follows:

- Mesoglow: Weekly sessions for 1 month followed by monthly maintenance
- Mesoglow with hydration:
  - Phase 1: initialize, four sessions at weekly intervals
  - Phase 2: repair, two sessions monthly
  - Phase 3: maintain, one session every 2–6 months
- Mesolift with hyaluronic acid: three sessions, once in 2 weeks and then maintenance once in 3/6 months.

In facial rejuvenation, cocktails of glutathione, vitamin C, organic silicium, and hyaluronic acid have been used with reasonable success and the author himself has experience of using these products for patients of dry skin, wrinkles, and hyperpigmentation

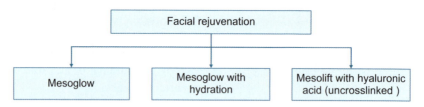

Flowchart 1: Varieties of facial rejuvenation.

TABLE 1: Recommendations of facial rejuvenation mesotherapies			
	Mesoglow	**Mesoglow with hydration**	**Mesolift with hyaluronic acid**
Age	35 years	35–50 years	50 years
Dryness	–	Mild–moderate	Severe
Dullness	+	+	+
Wrinkles	–	+	+ +

(as a second/third line treatment). Readymade cocktails of the above mentioned products are available, but should not be confused with products which are meant to be used with iontophoresis or needleless mesotherapy machines (the latter should not be injected).

A good cocktail for facial rejuvenation, especially for young patients, would be gluthatione, vitamin C, organic silicium and sodium taurinate in the ratio of 1.3:0.5:0.3:0.3. For older patients with concerns of hydration and wrinkling, hyaluronic acid (uncrosslinked) can be added to the above mentioned in a quantity of 2 mL. All these need to be injected intradermally, either manually or with the help of a mesogun (Figure 2).

Injecting these cocktails provides support and essential elements for normal skin turnover and repair. It also stimulates collagen and hyaluronic acid production, inhibits melanin, promotes microcirculation and protects from free radical damage. It can also give gratifying results in cases of postacne hyperpigmentation and scars (Figures 3 and 4).

For cellulite reduction, readymade cocktails are preferred in Mesotherapy. Deep injections of phosphatidyl choline/deoxycholate called Injection lipolysis are not to be confused with it. In June 2015, the Food and Drug

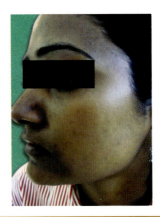

Figure 3: Facial rejuvenation in a patient with postacne hyperpigmentation (before).

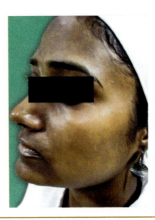

Figure 4: Facial rejuvenation in a patient with postacne hyperpigmentation (after 4 weekly sessions of glutathione + vitamin C + sodium taurinate + organic silicium).

Administration has approved deoxycholic acid[2] for use in submental fat reduction. Readymade cocktails for mesotherapy contain caffeine and hyaluronic acid and act by a mechanism of improving blood flow to the cellulite area, dissolving excess fat deposits, removing fibrotic, hardened connective tissue and improving lymphatic drainage (Figure 5).

For hair loss therapy, a plethora of products are available. Dutasteride, finasteride,

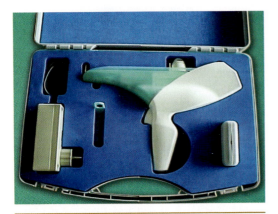

Figure 2: Mesogun with guard, charger and battery.

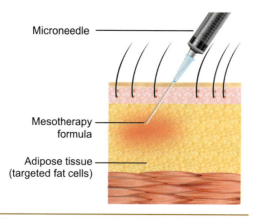

Figure 5: Mesotherapy for cellulite reduction.

This treatment is an adjunct to conventional medical treatment and serves as a bridge between medical and surgical options. Dermarollers have been used at times with these cocktails where a mesogun is unavailable. Manual intradermal injections can be done but are more painful. Indications are mainly chronic telogen effluvium and androgenetic alopecia (Hamilton Norwood up to type 3 and Ludwig up to type 2) (Figures 6 and 7).

Choice of patients for whom the authors would recommend mesotherapy is very important as this is one science wherein small doses are distributed over large areas.

minoxidil, biotin, dexpanthenol, *Gingko biloba*, etc. have been used as mesotherapy drugs. Recommended cocktails are:
- Readymade cocktails (mixture of vitamins)—5 mL
- Minoxidil 5% + haircare—1 mL each
- Minoxidil 5% + dexpanthenol—1 mL each
- Minoxidil 5% + dexpanthenol + biotin + *Gingko biloba*—0.5 mL each
- Finasteride/dutasteride (0.3 mL) + procaine 1 mL.

Sessions are done weekly for 6 weeks, followed by 6 sessions every 2 weeks, followed by maintenance every month. Patients are advised to wash scalp with an antibacterial shampoo on the day of treatment and the day after. Preprocedure thorough cleaning is done with spirit and povidone iodine. Multiple injections are done over the frontal, temporal and vertex areas of the scalp using the mesogun. Medicines are delivered at a depth of 4 mm.

Hair stops falling in 2–4 weeks. Regrowth can be seen as early as 4–6 weeks. Treatment necessary indefinitely as stopping treatment leads to reversion to the pretreatment balding pattern. Ideally, if treatment with minoxidil is commenced as soon as hair loss becomes apparent, the need for surgical treatment can be prevented.

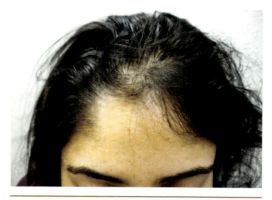

Figure 6: Before Mesotherapy

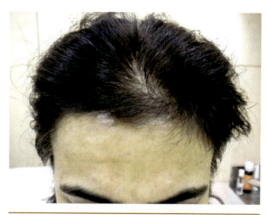

Figure 7: After 6 sessions of mesotherapy with readymade cocktails of vitamins

❑ ADVANTAGES

It has advantages, such as:
- Quick, office procedure
- Can be done under local anesthesia
- Little down time
- Suitable for all skin types
- Side effects are minimal
- No scars
- Safe as long as the procedure is performed by a well-trained medical practitioner who adheres to strict infection control and hygiene.

❑ CONTRAINDICATIONS

Contraindications for mesotherapy are:
- Allergy to ingredients
- History of hypertrophic scars
- Bleeding abnormalities
- Pregnancy and lactation
- Autoimmune disorders (lupus and scleroderma)
- Epilepsy
- Diabetes (uncontrolled)
- Herpes simplex virus 1 (under the cover of antivirals)
- Inflammatory skin disorders
- Patients on oral isotretinoin, oral steroids and immunosuppressants
- Unrealistic expectations
- Active bacterial infection at the treatment site.

In facial rejuvenation, patients who are looking for instant and short-term gratifying results and ready to do repeat sessions are the ideal candidates. It does not replace either botulinum toxin, which is used for treating dynamic wrinkles or fillers, which are used to augment volume loss or treat static wrinkles. It can work in tandem with fractional resurfacing devices and improve the hydration and the texture of the skin.

Some of the disadvantages are:
- Only for mild-to-moderate aging
- Mild erythema and burning postinjections
- Small hematomas
- Possibility of allergic reactions
- Lack of controlled clinical trials
- Lack of guidelines.

In the case of cellulite reduction, patients with excessive amount of fat are not ideal candidates. It can be used for young patients who exercise regularly, but have pockets of cellulite over their hips and thighs. This can be used as a follow-up treatment postliposuction or even injection lipolysis or in combination with fat reduction devices that involve cryolipolysis or use radiofrequency. Monthly sessions, from 4–6, are required for optimum results.

In hair loss treatment, be it telogen effluvium or androgenetic alopecia, the first line of treatment is medical therapy. Mesotherapy can be used to fast track the treatment as it helps in cutting down the hair loss and, therefore, alleviates the patient's anxiety. Cocktails containing dutasteride, biotin, caffeine, etc. can be used weekly for up to six sessions to reduce hair loss.

❑ COMPLICATIONS

Mesotherapy has had both its advocates and detractors. Amin et al. found no significant clinical or histologic changes after multivitamin mesotherapy for skin rejuvenation. The conclusion was that multivitamin and hyaluronic acid solution facial mesotherapy does not appear to provide any significant benefit.[3]

On the other hand, Lacarubba et al. concluded that mesotherapy with hyaluronic acid may be an effective treatment for skin photoaging, as confirmed by ultrasound. Not all patients respond uniformly to hyaluronic acid and some may not respond at all.[4]

Duque-Estrada et al. reported two cases of patchy alopecia that developed after mesotherapy for the treatment of androgenetic alopecia. In the first patient, alopecia developed after injections of the heparinoid vasodilator mesoglycan; the 3-month follow-up examination revealed a small residual area of cicatricial alopecia. The second patient developed reversible alopecia after multiple scalp injections of homeopathic agents.[5]

With its increased popularity, there has been an increase in the number of reported side effects resulting from mesotherapeutic intervention. Kadry et al. reported multifocal scalp abscesses with subcutaneous fat necrosis as a direct result of mesotherapy; therefore, requiring extensive surgical repair.[6]

Venkataram concluded that data on its safety and efficacy in pattern hairloss have not been adequately and critically evaluated and documented in proper, peer-reviewed clinical trials.[7]

Since its description by Michael,[8] mesotherapy has had turbulent times with very little by way of literature to prove its efficacy though clinically physicians who practice it can vouch for it. It still is a gray area but a science worth exploring, especially in situations where therapeutics have fared badly or failed like hair loss, facial rejuvenation and cellulite reduction.

❏ CONCLUSION

Mesotherapy is still in its evolutionary phase. It is unpredictable in its efficacy with variable results. It is considered exotic among many dermatologists. Its most popular use remains facial rejuvenation. In all of the indications, it remains a second line of therapy and because of its expense, large scale use has not occurred.

❏ REFERENCES

1. Conseil d'État: Ordonnance du 17 juin 2011, SARL Cellusonic et autres, Madame Valérie A et autres.
2. FDA News Release—FDA approves treatment for fat below the chin. 29th April 2015.
3. Amin SP, Phelps RG, Goldberg DJ. Mesotherapy for facial skin rejuvenation: A clinical, histologic and electron microscopic evaluation. Dermatol Surg. 2006;32: 1467-72.
4. Lacarrubba F, Tedeschi A, Nardone B, Micali G. Mesotherapy for skin rejuvenation: Assessment of the subepidermal low echogenic band by ultrasound evaluation with cross-sectional B-mode scanning. Dermatol Ther. 2008;21: S1-5.
5. Duque-Estrada B, Vincenzi C, Misciali C, Tosti A. Alopecia secondary to mesotherapy. J Am Acad Dermatol. 2009;61(4):707-9.
6. Kadry R, Hamadah I, Al-Issa A, Field L, Alrabiah F. Multifocal scalp abscess with subcutaneous fat necrosis and scarring alopecia as a complication of scalp mesotherapy. J Drugs Dermatol. 2008;7(1):72-3.
7. Mysore V. Mesotherapy in management of hairloss - Is it of any use? Int J Trichology. 2010;2(1):45-6.
8. Pistor M. What is mesotherapy? Chir Dent Fr. 1976;46: 59-60.

Monopolar Radiofrequency: Ways to Handle Complications

Simal Soin, Anusha H Pai

❏ INTRODUCTION

Radiofrequency (RF) has been traditionally used in healthcare applications for years together. Over a period of time, technologies have been utilized better to offer enhanced efficacy along with safety to the clients.

The RF applications are based on two basic principles:

1. Monopolar RF: the single electrode on the applicator tip emits microcurrents to the treatment area through suitable medium like oil or gel. The current passes through the body to the return pad connected remotely on the body areas. Through the return pad, currents are taken back to the device completing the loop. Due to the remote placement of return pad, the current signal penetrates deeper producing substantial heat to achieve desired results

2. Bipolar RF: unlike monopolar, in bipolar both the current emitting electrode and the return earthing electrodes are available on the applicator tip itself. Due to the close associated electrodes, currents usually flow over the tip itself completing short loop. This results in minimal penetration of the signals producing superficial heating of the skin. Indications such as skin rejuvenation, fine lines, and skin laxity can be nicely addressed with bipolar.

Monopolar RF is used for tightening the face, eyes, neck, crepey skin, abdomen, flanks, back rolls, thighs, calves, hands, upper arms, and breast lift. It is a very comfortable treatment with no down time. During the treatment, the client feels a warm sensation and can resume to normal daily activity after the treatment. Sometimes slight redness can occur which usually subsides in an hour or two.

❏ TECHNOLOGIES IN RADIOFREQUENCY DEVICES

There are two types of technologies in RF devices:

1. Monopolar static RF (Thermage Thermacool device): it is a great tool for contouring and skin tightening by virtue of the strong collagen remodeling it causes. The result peaks at 4–6 months but with the newer machines, the results are quicker. The limitation is the inability to treat the neck with adequate energies because of the lack of fatty tissue in the neck. The heat tends to be too intense making the treatment uncomfortable and painful. The

hooding and wrinkling around the eye area can be treated. This is referred to as a nonsurgical blepharoplasty. Abdomen can be treated with a large tip. This device works well in older people with a very lax skin or in older people with a strong/large double chin. For younger patients, it provides a good contouring[1]

2. Monopolar RF in motion (BTL Exilis Elite): this requires about four sessions on the face to see an appreciable result. With every session there will be a perceptible improvement. There is no limit to the number of sessions that can be done provided the malar fat is not tampered with since it needs to be preserved. It works well on younger and older patients with square faces. Multiple sessions can improve the squaring of the face.

Monopolar RF devices in motion used for body treatment uses a combination of 3.2 MHz of monopolar RF with ultrasound energy which causes a substantial improvement on body circumference through fat lipolysis and skin tightening at the same time. It delivers high energy to different layers of the skin and fat as a result of which fat reduction and skin tightening occurs at the same time.

❑ MECHANISM OF ACTION OF MONOPOLAR RADIOFREQUENCY

The simplest way to describe the mechanism of monopolar RF is that it is heat that gets delivered into the collagen in the dermis and fibrous septa in the subcutaneous fat. The body perceives the heat as a wound and remodels the collagen. As a result of collagen remodeling, the skin gets firmer, tighter, lifted, and contoured. The result is a rested, fresher, and less tired look.

When combined with the ultrasound energy, the fat cells are heated to a temperature

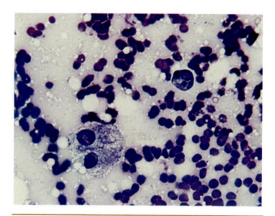

Figure 1: Apoptosis.

at which they are destroyed (apoptosis) and are eliminated through the lymphatic system (Figure 1). The thermal energy simultaneously encourages the production of new and firmer collagen which tightens the skin.[2,3]

The results lasts long time for up to 1 year depending on the slackening and sagging of the skin. Lifestyle modification is required for the body treatment results to last for a long time. The fillers last longer post monopolar RF skin tightening.

The complications associated with the technology/treatments can be broadly categorized in three major segments.

1. Client related
2. Product related
3. Environment related.

Client Related Complications

Criteria for selecting the right candidate:
- While treating the candidates for nonsurgical body shaping, fat lipolysis, and skin tightening, it is very important for us to choose the right candidates meeting the criteria of selection (Figure 2)
- Body mass index (BMI) is a simple tool for defining obesity. Candidates with BMI less than 28 can show significant improvement with noninvasive body contouring. Obese

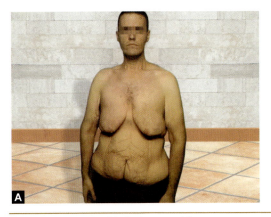
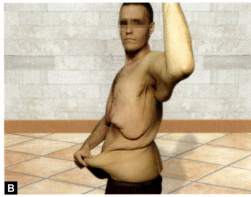

Figure 2: Excessive skin laxity—avoid.

patients with BMI more than 30 are often not good candidates for noninvasive body contouring and may require diet, bariatric, or other surgical interventions (Figure 3)

- Clients older than 40 years tend to develop dry skin due to lower hydration levels in the body. This could lead to slower results due to suboptimal collagen fibers in the body. Heat generated in the treatment area by the device has limitation in creating neocollagenesis, showing slower results. These clients should be prescribed with good moisturizer to be applied three times a day. Drinking 3–4 liters of water per day can significantly enhance the hydration of the skin. This ensures adequate drainage of apoptotic fat cells through the lymphatics
- Clients who smoke and drink can also have unsatisfactory results. Better hydration levels built up during the treatment periods can enhance the results significantly
- Candidates with busy schedule are the most difficult cases to satisfy. Various treatment protocols for different body areas with multiple sessions can be spaced out for such patients. Missing the sessions at the preset duration time could compromise results. It is evident that the client must complete the prescribed sessions according to protocols to get a satisfactory result

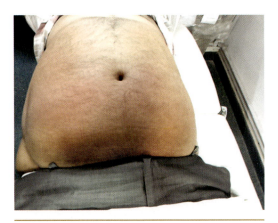

Figure 3: Avoid if body mass index more than 28.

- Client motivation is another vital parameter for achieving amazing outcomes at the end of few sessions
- Patient counseling is very important. It is of prime importance for the doctor to analyze the patient and set the right expectations. Treatment should not be undertaken in people with predominantly tight visceral fat.

Product Related Complications

- It is very important for a successful practice to choose good technology with Food and

Drug Administration certification. Using nonbranded, noncertified devices can lead to lot of complications building more and more unhappy clientele. The results from monopolar RF devices are steady but not as dramatic as surgery

- Sensitive areas with thin skin should be treated with caution, such as the medial thighs and upper arms, because erythema can last much longer and there is a possibility of minor burns or blistering over areas where there is sweating or the loss of tip contact of the handpiece

- Excessive heat with high pressures on the treatment areas can lead to "panniculitis". Panniculitis is sudden necrosis of the fat cell.[4] Refining the application technique can evade the possibility of panniculitis among the clients. In case of its occurrence, mild thumb massage on the lump can help dissolve it gradually. Slight pain associated with panniculitis can be managed by taking some oral anti-inflammatory/pain tablets

- Monopolar devices usually incorporate disposable return pads. Usage of damaged pad can lead to mild blisters at the return pad application area due to direct conductivity of the microcurrents from the skin to metal electrode (Figure 4)

- The quicker the impact to the treatment area in terms of heat generation, the better the results tend to be. Prolonging the heat generation with low power exposures can lead to activation of heat shock proteins preventing apoptosis and thereby good results

- Usage of gel or oil not recommended by the manufacturer during the treatments can lead to unpleasant heat experience and also allergies on the treatment areas of sensitive skin.

Environment Related Complications

- Improper cooling in the treatment room can lead to sweating during the treatment creating Arching or superficial burns due to reaction of sweat with RF signals. Ensure adequate cooling in the treatment room before and during the treatment for better comfort and tolerance by the client (Figure 5)

- Patient's bed/couch plays important role in client comfort. Flexible couch with up/down and front/back movements can help position client in appropriate posture to treat conveniently by the therapist. Sufficient space around the couch helps therapist move freely around the client while treating different body areas.

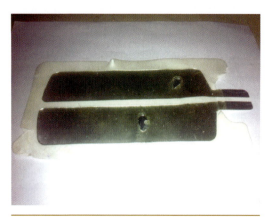

Figure 4: Defective return pad.

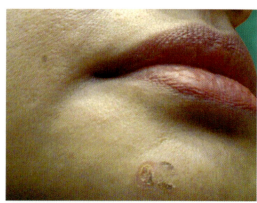

Figure 5: Superficial burn.

❏ CONCLUSION

Monopolar radiofrequency is without a doubt the finest, safest, and most effective noninvasive, nonsurgical modality for treating laxity of the face and other areas of the body. The deep penetration and combination of ultrasound and RF causing apoptosis is the key to its success. The few important prerequisites for obtaining the best results are good hydration levels, good training (since the procedure is operator dependent), and good patient selection.

❏ REFERENCES

1. Sukhal SA, Geronemus RG. Thermage: the nonablative radiofrequency for rejuvenation. Clin Dermatol. 2008;26(6): 602-7.
2. Zelickson B, Ross EV, Strasswimmer J. Definition and proposed mechanisms of non-invasive skin tightening. In: Alam M, Dover J, editors. Non-surgical skin tightening and lifting. Philadelphia: Elsevier; 2009. p. 3-7.
3. Alster, TS, Lupton JR. Nonablative cutaneous remodeling using radiofrequency devices. Clin Dermatol. 2007;25:487-91.
4. Zelickson BD, Kist D, Bernstein E, Brown DB, Ksenzenko S, Burns J, et al. Histological and ultrastructural evaluation of the effects of a radiofrequency based non-ablative dermal remodeling device: a pilot study. Arch Dermatol. 2004;140:204-9.

Complications in Bipolar Radiofrequency Therapy

Narmada Matang

❑ INTRODUCTION

Radiofrequency (RF) electric energy has a history of over 70 years in the field of medicine. The term RF energy applies because the oscillation frequency of the current is in the broadcasting band of the electromagnetic spectrum. Radiofrequency has been in use for cauterization in multiple applications and today, it is indeed one of the most promising mode of treatment for not only for improvement of facial rhytides and wrinkles but also acne, scars, open pores, stretch marks, treatment for excessive sweating and facial or body contouring.

Radiofrequency systems work on the principle of controlled thermal heating where resistance in the target tissue to the RF current creates electrothermal damage; the higher the level of the current, the greater the damage. Earlier external RF systems, where electrodes are placed on the skin, appeared first; "unipolar" RF, where a single delivery electrode was placed over the target tissue and a return electrode was placed elsewhere;

and "bipolar" RF, where the delivery and return electrodes were combined in a single handpiece. These systems had problems with accurate depth delivery, necessitated multiple treatments to get any noticeable effect, and required aggressive cooling to protect the epidermis from electrothermal damage. Further research led to development of technologies with noninsulated and insulated microneedles which could deliver precise zones of fractionated electrothermal damage with minimal downtime fast recovery and excellent results (Figure 1).

Some common terms used in RF are discussed below:
- Monopolar RF: RF energy is delivered with only the delivery electrode, the return electrode is fixed elsewhere on the body. The RF energy travels outwards from the electrode in a fan-shaped pattern as it seeks out the return electrode
- Bipolar RF: here, the delivery and return electrodes are mounted in the handpiece. The depth of penetration of the electric

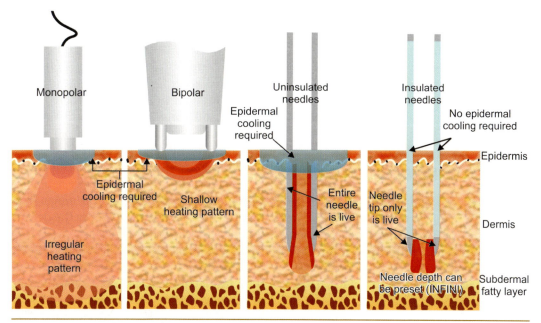

Figure 1: Various techniques of delivering radiofrequency energy.

current as it passes between the electrodes is limited to one-half of the distance between the electrodes

- Fractionated RF with uninsulated microneedles: the depth problem is solved, but because of the entire needle shaft comprising the electrode, the electrothermal damage is delivered down the whole needle, thus also requiring epidermal cooling

- Fractionated RF with insulated microneedles: the needle is insulated except for the very tip, no electrothermal damage is delivered to either the epidermis or the insulated area of the needle above the tip. This way, RF can be used to generate fractional zones of coagulation not just mild reversible denaturation

- External RF devices rely on the skin thickness, hydration, and the composition of collagen and fat which can lead to placement of the energy at an unknown or variable depths. The variation in the target

level of energy can lead to fat necrosis if deep and or burns and post-inflammatory hyperpigmentation if superficial. An important factor is achieving adequate tissue temperature for appropriate tissue wound healing response and collagen production. Multiple treatments are hence required for appreciable results as collagen stimulation is limited with single treatment. Most of the cutaneous RF devices have an issue of unpredictable heating and hence inadequate results and this is an underlying challenge to understand and customize each patient on tolerance and visible inflammatory response for visible results.[1]

Recent advances to ablative technology is the fractionated RF technology which creates a low density fractional epidermal and superficial dermal coagulation under conductive pins and delivers RF energy through the reticular dermis combining a low density ablative effect in the epidermis and subnecrotic heating in the deeper layers of skin.[2] This fractionated approach, with relatively low impact epidermal junctional effect and deep dermal effect, has been coined as the fractional sublative resurfacing. Multiple nonaggressive treatment sessions have shown improvement in fine lines acne scars and tissue tightening.[3]

❏ CLINICAL INDICATIONS

Let us look at clinical indications of this technology, with the novel approach of low intensity fractionated RF, many skin concerns can be addressed and have been published already.

- Active acne
- Acne scars
- Improvement of skin texture—open pores and fine lines
- Skin tightening and contouring
- Striae
- Excessive sweating.

Inflammatory Acne

Nonablative RF devices have also been used effectively for the treatment of moderate to severe inflammatory acne vulgaris. It has been suggested that the mechanism of action of nonablative RF is mainly a reduction of sebaceous gland activity and the promotion of dermal architecture remodeling by thermal stimulation. The mechanism of action of these devices is thought to be related to the fact that water, collagen, melanin, and dermal microvasculature absorb RF energy, producing a bulk heating effect on the dermis and inducing cellular mediator and growth factor secretion, which results in wound healing.[4]

Ruiz-Esparza and Gomez demonstrated that nonablative RF can also be used as a safe and effective treatment for moderate to severe acne vulgaris. According to their report, an

excellent response was noted in more than 80% of participants who underwent nonablative RF treatments, and no remarkable side effects were detected.[5] The authors suggested that thermal stimulation produced by the RF-based system seemed to inhibit sebaceous gland activity and stimulate dermal architecture remodeling, resulting in clinical improvement in the inflammatory acne lesions.[5]

Hantash et al. first demonstrated the effects of the minimally invasive RF device, a bipolar microneedle electrode system, on human skin. They created RF thermal zones in the dermis using microneedle electrode pairs.[6]

In the study conducted by Sang Lee et al., the microneedle device used did not have insulated needles and this has the risk of epidermal damage, however, no such side effect was observed. With a calculated risk, one can avoid such adverse effects. In fact if the energy levels are appropriate, then one can observe a good textural improvement as well.[7]

Acne Scars

Fractionated RF results in volumetric heating and heat diffusion to deeper level and the skin needling with microneedles has been reported to stimulate migration and proliferation of keratinocytes and fibroblasts by inducing several growth factors.[8] Regeneration and realignment of irregular and thick collagen bundles through physical breakage because of the holes made into the skin by needles eventually leads to clinically better scar and texture.[9]

Acne scars are commonly encountered clinical scene in a regular dermatology and cosmetic consultations. Acne scars are visible resolution to deep inflammation as a consequence of acne. It can be a result of superficial acne but more often associated with nodulocystic acne. A study showed that 16% of patients with acne seek proper treatment and among those seeking medical advice, 74% wait greater than 12 months for therapy of their acne.[10]

Atrophic scarring appears to be commonly associated with acne. The major clinical types of atrophic scars are ice pick, rolling and box, or depressed fibrotic scars.[11,12]

Skin Rejuvenation: Improvement of Skin Texture

Fractionated microneedle RF treats the texture of the skin at epidermal level thus improving the texture of the skin making it more smoother with less visible open pores and fine lines through the wound healing process.

In a study by Hruza et al.,[13] subjects who received fractional RF treatments showed clinical improvement in skin texture by investigators' assessment, which was greater than 40%. In another study regarding facial photodamage in Asians, fractional RF treatments produced moderate (26–50%) and incremental improvements in skin smoothness and tightness.[14] These results of previous studies in clinical improvement of overall skin appearance are comparable with those of our study, which shows 26–75% improvement over baseline. In particular, this is the first study using microneedle fractional RF, to our knowledge, which showed statistically significant improvement both in degree of skin roughness measured by visiometer and in histologic quantitative assessment of procollagen-1. In addition, erythema and melanin index showed improvement but without statistical significance.[15]

Skin Tightening and Contouring

It is an extended application of skin rejuvenation in terms of skin tightening or rather reduction in skin laxity that this technology can be applied for the purpose of facial contouring and skin tightening post certain surgical procedures like liposuction of larger body parts. While reduction in skin laxity has been published, there are not many documented studies on contouring. The author has used the technology for facial and body contouring as well, however, one should be careful for the choice of client and expectation alignment of the final outcome after multiple treatments. The technology has been used by the author for facial contouring of the lower face especially after injectable lipolysis. As also for cellulite treatment for the thighs and contouring of the arms postliposuction. In fact, many patients develop uneven appearance after the liposuction procedure and with careful examination and calculation of which areas need to be given more number of passes it can be addressed to satisfactory even result.[16]

Striae

Striae distensae are atrophic linear dermal scars with epidermal atrophy which occurs as a result of excessive dermal stretching. There have been some reports of microneedle fractional RF being used for treatment of striae.[17,18]

Excessive sweating recent reports have suggested that fractional microneedle RF can be used for effectively treating the axillary hyperhydrosis. However, there are no published reports of the same.

❑ WHICH PATIENTS YOU WOULD AVOID AND WHY

In the author's experience, cosmetic consultation are always very intense and detailed as the physicians deals with very healthy and demanding patients who have high expectation from the services offered, yet it should not have downtime or adverse effects. While they should be able to notice considerable visible results no one should know about treatments!

While bipolar microneedle RF is relatively safe procedure, results can be compromised in individuals with other medical issues like diabetes or immunological disorders.

Hence, the following types of patients should be avoided:

- Patient with very high expectations and limited patience: these are difficult to deal with and will always expect more in less time, sometimes the effort that goes into convincing them is much more than the efforts required in performing the services; hence at least initially, it is better to avoid such patients
- Keloidal tendency: it is important to take an informed consent of the possibility of the risk that both the patient and the performing doctor are taking though keloids on face are rare it is mandatory to discuss the possible consequences with the patient. It is indeed patients right to know the risk involved
- Patient on isotretinoin: isotretinoin makes the skin extremely sensitive and dry, it is better to avoid and wait for a washout period of at least 2 months before starting this service
- Pregnancy: many hormonal changes are taking place inside the body which may influence the outcome, hence always better to wait and counsel the patient. There are no studies to prove the safety of such procedures in case of any adverse event as well
- Concurrent systemic diseases or immunosuppression hematologic diseases with bleeding tendency or diabetes mellitus and atopic dermatitis: all these conditions affect the wound healing process which can compromise the final result.

- Currently taking anticoagulants or antiplatelet agents: while one can take such patients, it would always be safe to take an informed consent and align the patient about some minor bleeding points which can be controlled
- Previous history of frequent herpes simplex viral infection of the face: simply for possibility of activation of such infection
- Aesthetic procedures on the face: heat can hasten the biodegradation of temporary filler if procedure is performed in the same area, hence history taking is important for scheduling the treatment
- Any implantable electronic device: e.g., pacemaker
- Previous history of hypersensitivity to anesthetic creams: while this may sound simple to deal with, it can be quite an issue to deal with in darker skin type with risk of postinflammatory hyperpigmentation. Patients can be very unforgiving if they develop any adverse consequence due to procedure!

Procedure (Figure 2)

Following are the steps to be followed for performing the procedure:

- Consultation and alignment rule out all contraindications during consultation
- Consent form to be signed
- Photo documentation
- Planning on areas of concern and number of passes
- Local anesthetic cream application on concern area
- Starting the service as per the plan.

Treatment Protocol

- Step 1: after complete removal of the anesthetic cream with normal saline, repeat cleansing with a good cleanser in case of inflammatory acne or 70% alcohol if there is no inflammation

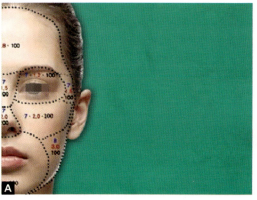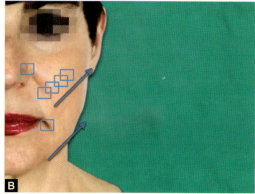

Figure 2: Treatment zones and overlap tip placement while treating the concern areas.

- Step 2: load the sterile tip on to the handpiece as per the manual instructions. Start the treatment holding the handpiece perpendicular to the skin, keep a sterile gauze piece in case of some pinpoint bleeding especially in case of active inflammatory acne

- Step 3: generally all devices have manuals which has protocols and guidelines for depth of the needle and it is indeed a good idea to follow them at the start especially during the first session. However, during subsequent sessions, one can just look for some erythema as a guidance along with patient tolerance to the heat. One important point is to make sure the technique is stamping and one must wait for the needle disc to move up before you move ahead this is to avoid the scratch marks which can happen if the hand piece has moved before the needles have come up and out

- Step 4: set the control panel on depth power and speed as per plan start with less penetration depth and then increase as per tolerance and local tissue reaction. About 100–150 shots would cover one half of the face. Repeat the procedure in similar manner 3–4 times. In case of excessive erythema or edema, shift to the other side

and come back to the same side once the redness has settled. This is to avoid any remote chances of postinflammatory hyperpigmentation

- Step 5: work across the face starting from the upper neck upwards in a crisscross manner against gravity. Stamping perpendicular to the static rhytides is advised. Stamping method with a 50% overlap and 2–3 passes is advised. After completing the session, cold compression is soothing for the patient. Apply mild moisturizer soon after and a thick layer of sunscreen before the patient leaves the treatment room figure 3.

Tips

- Generally start with 6–7 power because as the tissue heats up it may not be feasible to give high energy at subsequent passes. The depth of the needle at the first session is strictly according to the protocols given in the manual. During the second and later sessions, increase the depth by 1 mm all over depending on the patient tolerance, keeping an eye on local tissue reaction

- All the movement of the stamping are upwards starting from the neck area to forehead. In case of acne, 500–600 shots

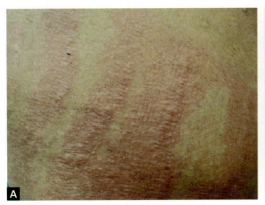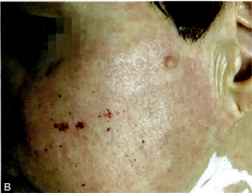

Figure 3: Mild erythema to pin point bleeding may be noticed while performing the procedure, which disappears in couple of hours.

are given on the affected areas and the rest to the normal or unaffected area for overall oil control or textural improvement. The author generally concentrates on the jawline and upper neck as it give good tightening effect in case of laxity of skin and the patients are quite satisfied with the change. The author generally finishes 900–1,000 shots in about 45 minutes and never uses the same tip again for the same client. Patients tolerate the procedure very well, in fact in the author's experience, patients closed to filler injections are right candidates for the skin tightening effects of bipolar RF. For each half of the face, 450–500 shots can be given at one sitting. Patient can be followed up for the next session after 4 weeks

- Concerns like periorbital laxity and eyebrow drooping can also be dealt with by repeated low energy passes around the region
- Striae: multiple passes with high energy works well a cocktail of vitamin C and HUA application within the passes is advisable
- Acne: control the bleeding in case of inflammatory acne with a sterile gauze, put the patient on antibiotics for 3 days postprocedure to control infection if any figures 4 to 9.

Complications

Just like any other technology, this technology also has some potential complications that can be very disturbing. This is otherwise a safe and easy technology to work with primarily because it is color blind. It is more tissue resistance, so depending on the tolerance of the patient, one has to customize the protocols in terms of depth of the needle and energy levels. Potential complications are mostly the result of overheating.

Burns

Possibility of thermal burns cannot be ruled out while performing bipolar fractionated needle RF this is due to epidermal damage that may appear as tiny blisters on the skin surface after the procedure. It is important to align the patient that in case of discomfort or sustained erythema, they should contact the performing doctor immediately.

Management

If such adverse event happens, it needs to be treated and managed as superficial thermal burns with oral and local steroids. It should

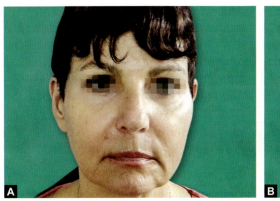
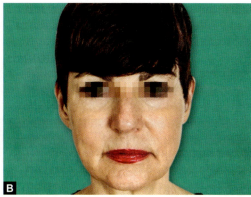

Figure 4: Facial rejuvenation and skin tightening in a 54-year-old patient after 4 monthly sessions of treatment.

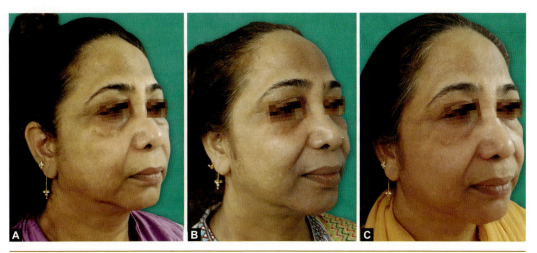

Figure 5: Facial skin tightening and contouring—mild improvement at the mentolabial and jowls seen after three sessions.

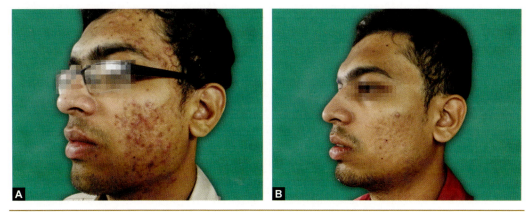

Figure 6: Active inflammatory acne can be treated with bipolar radiofrequency at monthly gaps two to three sessions give promising results.

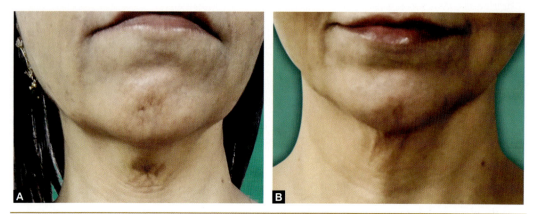

Figure 7: Neck skin laxity treated with single session of bipolar radiofrequency in a 57-year-old lady.

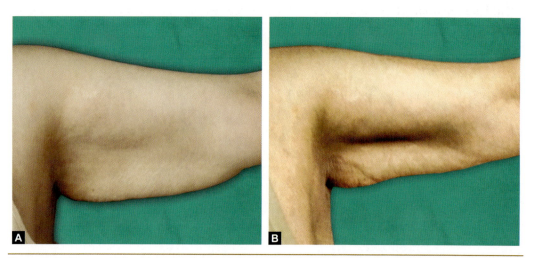

Figure 8: A 56-year-old female patient treated for skin laxity postliposuction procedure resulting in visible skin tightening and contouring after three sessions.

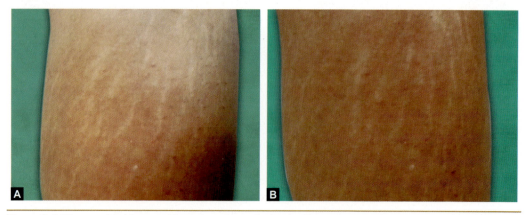

Figure 9: A 20-year-old girl treated for striae alba at the back of lower legs resulting in less visible striae after two sessions done month apart.

be kept in mind that thermal burns take long to heal and patients need to be aligned accordingly.

Underlying Melasma Trigger

This is a possibility due to overheating of the tissue, patient may not have any visible pigmentation, however, may develop soon after this treatment.

Management

Examination and history taking should be meticulous and any suspicion on the same should be covered in consent form while aligning. This can be avoided by keeping low energy with multiple passes, and cooling the epidermis while treating.

Postinflammatory Hyperpigmentation

This is a risk in the darker skin types, primarily because of the inflammation but is easy to manage figure 10.

Management

Control on tissue reaction by controlling the energy levels and or no of passes along with cooling this can be avoided. Strict sun protection with mild steroid application of a

couple of weeks can be advised in case this happens.

Linear Epidermal Breach or Scratch Marks

This is due to improper technique wherein before the needles have been retracted, the handpiece has moved leading to small cuts on the skin surface.

Management

While performing the procedure keep an eye on the hand movement. Keep the speed to low at the start and once comfortable increase the speed of the needle. If this happens treatment would be like managing postinflammatory hyperpigmentation.

❑ CONCLUSION

Bipolar RF is a promising technology which can be used for multiple indications. Patients are looking for minimally invasive yet effective results and this technology delivers the expected results. The results suggest that bipolar microneedling RF significantly improved the skin quality in elasticity sebum content, thus making it one of the choices for oily acne prone skin, active acne, fine lines and wrinkles, stretch

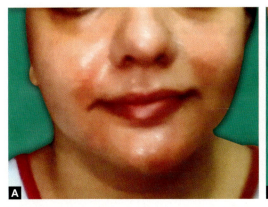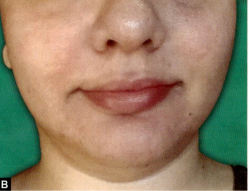

Figure 10: Adverse event of postinflammatory hyperpigmentation managed with mild local steroid application.

marks, and skin laxity. The procedure is well-tolerated by most of the patients with few side effects. Three to four sessions with an interval of 1 month suffices for desirable results and the maintenance can be planned once in 2–3 months. One can combine it with other services as well for customized results.

❑ REFERENCES

1. Weiner S. A review of radio frequency for skin tightening. Available from: http://www.international.lutronic.com/pdf/INFINI_WP_skin_tightening_Dr_Weiner.pdf.

2. Hruza G, Taub AF, Collier SL, Mulholland SR. Skin rejuvenation and wrinkle reduction using a fractional radio frequency system. J Drugs Dermatol. 2009;8(3):259-65.

3. Mulholland RS, Ahn DH, Kreindel M, Paul M. Fractional ablative radio-frequency resurfacing in Asian and Caucasian skin: a novel method for deep radio frequency fractional skin rejuvenation. Journal of Cosmetics, Dermatological Sciences and Applications. 2012;2:144-50.

4. Elsaie ML, Choudhary S, Leiva A, Nouri K. Nonablative radiofrequency for skin rejuvenation. Dermatol Surg 2010;36:577-89.

5. Ruiz-Esparza J, Gomez JB. Nonablative radiofrequency for active acne vulgaris: the use of deep dermal heat in the treatment of moderate to severe active acne vulgaris (thermotherapy): a report of 22 patients. Dermatol Surg. 2003;29:333-9.

6. Hantash BM, Renton B, Berkowitz RL, Stridde BC, Newman J. Pilot clinical study of a novel minimally invasive bipolar microneedle radiofrequency device. Lasers Surg Med. 2009;41:87-95.

7. Lee SJ, Goo JW, Shin J, Chung WS, Kang JM, Kim YK, et al. Use of fractionated microneedle radiofrequency for the treatment of inflammatory acne vulgaris in 18 Korean patients. Dermatol Surg. 2012;38(3):400-5.

8. Fabbrocini G, Fardella N, Monfrecola A, Proietti I, Innocenzi D. Acne scarring treatment using skin needling. Clin Exp Dermatol. 2009;34:874-9.

9. Cho SB, Lee SJ, Kang JM, Kim YK, Kim DH. The treatment of burn scar-induced contracture with the pinhole method and collagen induction therapy: a case report. J Eur Acad Dermatol Venereol. 2008;22(4):513-4.

10. Tan J, Vasey T, Fung K. Beleifs and perceptions of patients with acne. J Am Acad Dermatol. 2001;44:439-45.

11. Rivera A. Acne scarring: a review of current treatment modalities. J Am Acad Dermatol. 2008;59:659-76.

12. Jacob C, Dover J, Kaminer M. Acne scarring: a classification system and review of treatment options. J Am Acad Dermatol. 2001;45:109-17.

13. Hruza G, Taub AF, Collier SL, Mulholland SR. Skin rejuvenation and wrinkle reduction using a fractional radiofrequency system. J Drugs Dermatol. 2009;8:259-65.

14. Lee HS, Lee DH, Won CH, Chang HW, Kwon HH, Kim KH, et al. Fractional rejuvenation using a novel bipolar radiofrequency system in Asian skin. Dermatol Surg. 2011;37:1611-9.

15. Seo KY, Yoon MS, Kim DH, Lee HJ. Skin rejuvenation by microneedle fractional radiofrequency treatment in Asian skin: clinical and histological analysis. Lasers Surg Med. 2012;44(8):631-6.

16. Park J, Shin JU, Cho S, Lee JH. The use of microneedle fractional radio frequency system in wrinkle reduction and skin tightening.

17. Suh DH, Lee SJ, Lee JH, Kim HJ, Shin MK, Song KY. Treatment of striae distensae combined enhanced penetration platelet-rich plasma and ultra sound after plasma fractional radio frequency. J Cosmet Laser Ther. 2012;14(6):272-6.

18. Güngör S, Sayilgan T, Gökdemir G, Ozcan D. Evaluation of ablative and non-ablative laser in the treatment of striae dispense. Indian J Dermatol Venereol Leprol. 2014;80(5):409-12.

Practical Problems in Chemical Peels

Umashankar Nagaraju, Savitha AS

❏ INTRODUCTION

Chemical peeling is the application of a chemical agent to the skin which causes controlled destruction of a part of or the entire epidermis, with or without the dermis, leading to exfoliation and removal of superficial lesions, followed by regeneration of new epidermal and dermal tissues.[1]

Chemical peeling is one of the most common procedures performed on an outpatient department basis in a dermatologist's clinic. The history of chemical peels dates as far back as the Egyptians, who used various animal oils and alabaster to improve skin texture. True exfoliation of the skin was first introduced in 1903 by George MacKee who used phenol to treat acne scarring. In the 1930s, lay operators used phenol to remove wrinkles. It was during that time that peeling of the neck skin resulted in hypertrophic scarring. This scared many people away from chemical peel. Urkov, in 1946, introduced salicylic acid as a skin surface exfoliant. In 1961, Baker and Gordon developed a formula for phenol face peeling that is widely accepted and used today.

During the 1980s, there was a resurgence of interest in finding appropriate light- or medium-depth peel alternatives to the standard phenol solution. Brody (1986) advocated the use of trichloroacetic acid (TCA) for light- or medium-depth peels. Weiss et al. (1988) demonstrated that by using retinoic acid (retin-A) for 6 months or longer; one could achieve some resolution of the surface wrinkling and removal of actinic and pigmented solar keratoses.[2]

❏ INDICATIONS

Indications for chemical peels can be broadly classified as aesthetic and therapeutic indications as given in table 1.

TABLE 1: Indications for chemical peels	
Aesthetic	**Therapeutic**
Pigmentary disorders	Actinic keratosis
	Seborrheic keratosis
Acne	Warts
Superficial acne scars	Dermatosis papulosa nigra
Photodamaged skin	

❏ CONTRAINDICATIONS

In general, the following are the contraindications for chemical peeling (Table 2). Any specific contraindication will be dealt in the respective section.

❏ CLASSIFICATION OF CHEMICAL PEELS

The classification of peels according to the histological depth of necrosis is given in table 3.[4]

TABLE 2: Contraindications for chemical peeling	
Absolute	**Relative**
• Active herpes infection • Open wounds • Ehler Danlos (postpeeling healing will be delayed or compromised) • Systemic collagen vascular disease	• Keloid formation • History of herpes infection • Patients with active inflammation as seen in seborrheic, atopic dermatitis, irritant or allergic dermatitis, rosacea and psoriasis, may be at an increased risk for postoperative complications secondary to alterations in the skin's normal barrier function[3] • Unrealistic patient expectations • Physical inability to properly care for the face postoperatively • Telangiectases • Anticipation of inadequate photo protection because of job, vocation, or recreation

TABLE 3: Classification of peels according to histological depth of necrosis		
Type of peel	**Depth**	**Agents used**
Very superficial light peels	Necrosis up to the level of stratum corneum	TCA 10%, GA 30–50%, salicylic acid 20–30% Jessner's solution 1–3 coats Tretinoin 1–5%
Superficial light peels	Necrosis through the entire epidermis up to basal layer	TCA 10–30%, GA 50–70%, Jessner's solution 4–7 coats
Medium depth peels	Necrosis up to upper reticular dermis; initially, there is epidermal necrosis, papillary dermal edema, and lymphocytic infiltration followed by increased collagen production in following months	TCA 35–50%, GA 70% plus TCA 35%, 88% phenol unoccluded, Jessner's solution plus TCA 35%, solid CO_2 plus TCA 35%
Deep peels	Necrosis up to mid-reticular dermis	Baker-Gordon phenol peel

TCA, trichloroacetic acid; GA, glycolic acid; CO_2, carbon dioxide.

Superficial and medium depth peels are more suited for Indian skin and will be dealt in this chapter. It is better to avoid deep peels in Fitzpatrick skin type IV-VI due to risk of hyperpigmentation and scarring.

Factors Modifying Depth of Peel[5]

- Peeling agent and its concentration—as the concentration increases, the depth of the peel also increases. Concentration of peeling agent can vary with the brands and formulations of same agent
- Availability of free acid in solution
- Duration of application for α-hydroxyl acids like glycolic acid
- Method of application—rubbing the peel increases the depth compared to painting the skin
- Characteristics of patients skin—thick skin decreases the depth
- Vigorous degreasing enhances penetration
- Priming with low concentration of glycolic acid or tretinoin thins the stratum corneum enhancing the penetration.

❑ GENERAL PRINCIPLES FOR CHEMICAL PEELING

Patient Evaluation and Selection

The technique of chemical peel is fairly easily learned by the physician. But, it takes a great deal of experience to learn how the various skin types respond to the peel solutions. The most important consideration before a peel is the selection of the appropriate patient for the procedure. Detailed medical history, amount of sun exposure, tendency for keloids, and postinflammatory hyperpigmentation should be noted. Routine biochemical investigations are not required unless phenol is used. Any impairment of liver or kidney function would impair the excretion of phenol and potentially increase the concentration of phenol in the

bloodstream, which could result in cardiac irregularities and even death. Therefore, prior to peel with phenol is planned, **hemogram, urinalysis, liver and renal function tests, and electrocardiograph have to be carried out.** Photographic documentation before and after the procedure should be maintained.

Adequate time should be spent in counseling the patient about the nature of treatment, possible side effects, downtime if any, expected outcome, and about the need for multiple sessions and stressing on the requirement of absolute sun protection afterwards. Informed consent is imperative.

Patients who have history of herpetic infections should be prescribed prophylactic antivirals 2 days prior to the procedure and continued for 7–10 days until complete re-epithelialization occurs.

Priming the Skin

The process of preparing the skin for chemical peeling is called priming. Priming should be done 2–4 weeks prior to the procedure. Advantages of priming are:

- Ensures uniform penetration of the peeling agent
- Enhances healing and maintains the effects achieved with the chemical peel[6]
- Reduces postinflammatory pigmentation
- Detects intolerance to any agent
- Enforces patient compliance.[1]

Priming agents are hydroquinone (2–4%), tretinoin (0.025%), adapalene (0.1%), glycolic acid (6–12%), kojic acid, and azelaic acid. Hydroquinone is preferred when there is risk of hyperpigmentation.[7] Tretinoin is known to reduce healing time after resurfacing.

Safety Precautions before Peeling

The label on the bottle must be checked before applying the peel. The patient's head should be elevated to 45°. To avoid accidental spillage, the opened bottle or the soaked applicator should not be passed over the face. A syringe filled with water or saline should be kept ready for irrigation of the eyes in case of accidental spillage.[1]

Test Peel

Postauricular test peel may be useful in assessing the suitability of patients for chemical resurfacing and may be especially helpful in identifying patients at increased risk of postoperative pigmentary dyschromias and allergic reactions. Although a favorable test is reassuring, it does not guarantee a positive outcome following full-face resurfacing.[8]

Procedure

The required strength of the peeling agent is poured into a glass beaker and the neutralizing agent is also kept ready. Patient is asked to wash the face with soap and water to remove sebum, dirt, and grime. Contact lens should be removed before a peel. The patient is made to lie down at 45°. Hair is pulled back with a head band. The skin is then gently degreased with acetone. Degreasing the skin allows the hydrophilic peeling agents to penetrate easily. Sensitive areas like the inner canthus of the eyes and nasolabial folds are protected with petroleum jelly. The peeling agent is then applied either with a brush or cotton-tipped applicator or gauze. The chemical is applied quickly as cosmetic units on the entire face, beginning from the forehead, then the right cheek, nose, left cheek, and chin in that order. Feathering strokes are applied at the edges to blend with surrounding skin and prevent demarcation lines. The endpoint and neutralization of each peel will be discussed in the respective section. The skin is gently dried with gauze and the patient is asked to wash with cold water until the burning subsides. The face is patted dry and rubbing should be avoided.[1]

Postprocedure Care

Cold compresses or calamine lotion may be used to soothe the skin. Only bland water based moisturizers are to be used until peeling is complete. Sun exposure after the peel may cause postinflammatory hyperpigmentation. Patients are instructed to avoid excessive sun exposure and use broad-spectrum sunscreens. It is advisable to continue sun protection till the next sitting. Gel-based sunscreens and physical methods of sun protection are recommended for those prone to acne. To avoid postinflammatory hyperpigmentation and scarring in dark-skinned patients, it is important to avoid facial scrubs, depilatory creams, waxing, bleaching, microdermabrasion, and laser hair removal for at least 1 week before the procedure and 10–14 days after.

Individual Peels

Glycolic Acid

Glycolic acid (GA) is one of the commonly used peeling agents for therapeutic and cosmetic indications. Glycolic acid peels are commercially available as free acids, partially neutralized (higher pH), buffered, or esterified solutions.[9] They are available in various concentrations ranging from 20 to 70%. Fabbrocini, in 2009, classified glycolic peels as very superficial (30–50% GA, applied for 1–2 min); superficial (50–70% GA, applied for 2–5 min); and medium depth (70% GA, applied for 3–15 min).[10]

Indications

- Acne
- Acne scars
- Melasma
- Postinflammatory hyperpigmentation
- Photoaging
- Seborrhea.

Procedure

Priming the skin with hydroquinone, or topical retinoids, has been found to increase peel efficacy and reduce the risk of postinflammatory hyperpigmentation.[7] The standard procedure mentioned above is followed. It is always better to start with a low concentration (20% GA) and increase the concentration and application time during subsequent sessions. There should be a minimum interval of 2 weeks between two treatment sessions. Peel neutralization is extremely important and it depends on erythema seen. Glycolic acid is not self-neutralizing and remains aggressive until buffered. However, in dark skin, it may be difficult to appreciate erythema. In such cases, it is better to time the peel between 3–5 minutes and judge the desired endpoint depending on the time.[11] Neutralization is done with 10–15% of sodium bicarbonate solution and then washed off with water. If frosting is observed in any particular area before the set time or endpoint, it is important to neutralize the peel immediately. Peeling is repeated once every 15 days for 4–6 months until the desired result is achieved.[12,13]

Correlation between depth of peel and skin appearance:[14]

- No erythema—no peeling
- Spots of erythema—very superficial
- Patches of erythema—very superficial
- Widespread erythema—superficial
- Small superficial blisters—deep
- Frosting—too deep for an α-hydroxy acids peel.

Postpeel

Erythema, stinging sensation, sensation of pulling of facial skin, mild burning, and transient postinflammatory hyperpigmentation may occur.

Side Effects

- Unbuffered GA can cause epidermolysis, which presents as whitening and blisters (Figure 1), followed by scarring. Epidermolysis may also occur if the patient has used topical retinoids, anti-acne creams, or skin lighteners in days prior to the peel which has resulted in exfoliation. If these creams are used as priming agents, patients should be instructed to stop the creams in case of severe exfoliation.
- Rarely, hypopigmentation, persistent erythema, and flare-up of acne
- Postinflammatory hyperpigmentation
- Lines of demarcation
- Allergic reactions
- Milia.

Management of Complications

Pain and Burning Sensation

Cold compresses and ice packs have to be applied immediately till the burning sensation subsides symptoms. Topical calamine lotion soothes the skin. Topical steroids, such as hydrocortisone or fluticasone, are prescribed

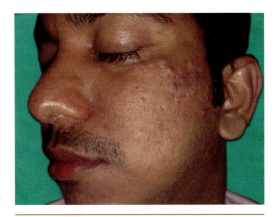

Figure 1: Whitening due to epidermolysis.

Photo courtesy: Dr Madan, Fellow of Cosmetic Dermatology, BMCRI to reduce the inflammation. Topical steroids may be continued once daily till symptoms subside (usually 2–3 days). Emollients moisturize the skin and sunscreens prevent postinflammatory hyperpigmentation.[15]

Hyperpigmentation

Fitzpatrick skin types III–VI are at increased risk for hyperpigmentation. Adequate priming of the skin with hydroquinone considerably reduces the risk of hyperpigmentation. Once hyperpigmentation develops retinoic acid, 0.05% cream in combination with 4% hydroquinone once or twice daily for 3 weeks or longer if necessary to be used. Hydrocortisone cream can be used for several weeks as needed if erythema due to retinoic acid poses a concern. Use of sunscreen with sun protection factor 30 to be advised.[16]

Persistent Erythema

It is characterized by the skin remaining erythematous beyond what is normal for an individual peel. Erythema disappears normally in 3–5 days in superficial peel, 15–30 days in medium peel, and 60–90 days in deep peel. It could be due to usage of topical tretinoin just before and after peel, isotretinoin administration (<0.5 mg/kg body weight) prior to peel, minimal amount of alcoholic beverages, contact dermatitis, contact sensitization, or exacerbation of pre-existing skin disease. Erythema is treated with topical, systemic, or intralesional steroids if thickening is occurring and pulsed dye laser to treat the vascular factors.[15]

Accidental Contact with the Eye

It is better to avoid peeling in the eyelids, especially upper eyelids. If peeling agent comes in contact with the eye, eye should be washed with plenty of water and artificial tears should be applied. If symptoms persist, specialist opinion should be taken.

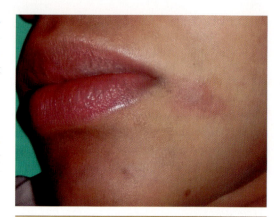

Figure 2: Erythema and blister formation with 50% glycolic acid.

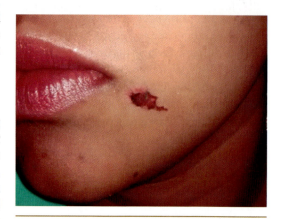

Figure 3: Scab formation after 4 days.

Photo courtesy: Dr Madan, Fellow of Cosmetic Dermatology, BMCRI

Blister and Scab Formation

If blisters are noted during the peel, the peel should be terminated immediately. Cool compresses and ice packs are given to reduce stinging. Hydrocortisone (1%) cream is prescribed. If reactions are severe, short course of systemic steroids, prednisolone 20–40 mg per day, single dose for 5 days can be given (Figures 2 and 3).

❏ COMBINATION TREATMENT[13]

Microneedling can be combined with 35% GA peel to treat acne scars. Microneedling is performed 6-weekly, and 35% GA peel 3 weeks after each microneedling session

- Glycolic acid and TCA peels are performed sequentially in cases of postinflammatory hyperpigmentation, postacne pigmentation, and melasma. This combination has been found to produce a deeper and more uniform peel than TCA used alone
- Combining Jessner's solution and GA for the treatment of photoaged skin, actinic keratoses, and rhytides resulted in a uniform GA peel, but the risk of over peel and scarring are high, especially in dark-skinned individuals[16]
- Glycolic acid has been combined with 5-fluorouracil to treat actinic keratosis. Pretreatment of the skin with 5-fluorouracil 5% increases the efficacy of the treatment and shortens the healing time[17]
- Glycolic acid peeling has also been used in combination with microdermabrasion, for the treatment of acne vulgaris and superficial acne scars, in order to increase treatment efficacy and achieve treatment goals within a shorter time. However, combining GA peels with microdermabrasion at the same session could lead to postinflammatory hyperpigmentation in skin types III–VI[12]
- Glycolic acid peeling is also combined with vitamin C in cases of melasma and postinflammatory hyperpigmentation
- Superficial GA peels can also be used with botulinum toxin and fillers in order to obtain overall improvement in wrinkles, skin tone, texture, radiance, and clarity. The peel was administered after injecting botulinum toxin during the same visit, or the procedures were separated by one or more days to minimize the potential for side effects.[18]

Lactic Acid

Lactic acid, also an α-hydroxy acid, has activities similar to GA, but milder. It has been found to be safe and an effective peeling agent for melasma in dark skin.[19] It is used as a peeling agent in its full strength of 92% and pH of 3.5. It also has a moisturizing effect. Lactic acid improves photodamaged skin and superficial pigmentation by inhibiting tyrosinase. Lactic acid is component of Jessner's peel.

Indications

- Dry skin
- Dyschromia
- Fine line
- For patients with sensitive skin and rosacea
- Melasma.[20]

Procedure

The standard procedure is followed and the endpoint determination and neutralization is similar to GA peel. The procedure can be repeated every 3 weeks for 4–5 sessions.

Side Effects

As lactic acid is a naturally occurring component on the skin, allergic reactions are minimal.

Salicylic Acid

Salicylic acid is derived from willow bark, wintergreen leaves and sweet birch.

Mechanism of Action

Salicylic acid is an excellent keratolytic agent. It is thought to function through solubilization of intercellular cement, thereby reducing corneocyte adhesion. Because of its lipophilic nature, salicylic acid has a strong comedolytic effect.[21]

Indications

- As salicylic acid is lipophilic, it is an ideal peeling agent for acne and seborrhea
- Acne
- Comedonal acne
- Rosacea

- Oily skin
- Enlarged facial pores
- Superficial acne scars
- Superficial pigmentary disorders like melasma
- Photoaged skin
- Freckles, lentigines.

Prepeel

When treating acne vulgaris, topical and systemic therapies (if indicated) are initiated 2–4 weeks prior to peeling. Topical antibiotics and benzoyl peroxide based products can be used daily and discontinued 1 or 2 days prior to peeling.[22]

Specific Contraindications

A history of allergy to aspirin.[23]

Procedure

Standard application procedure as mentioned above. The initial concentration is 20–30%, going up to 70%.[24] During application, the subject experiences a stinging and burning sensation which increases over the next 2 minutes, reaches a crescendo at 3 minutes, and then rapidly decreases to baseline over the next minute; this is considered the endpoint of the peel. As the hydroethanolic vehicle evaporates, it leaves behind a white precipitate of salicylic acid on the surface of the face which is termed as salicylic acid frost (Figure 4). This is pseudofrost unlike the frost which occurs due to coagulation of proteins. There is very little penetration of the active agent once the vehicle has volatilized. At this point, there is no burning or stinging as the agent causes a superficial anesthesia to light touch.[23] Face is washed with water and patted dry. Peels can be repeated once in 2 weeks for 5–6 sessions.

Postpeel

Patients report a tightness and smoothness immediately postpeel. Peeling usually

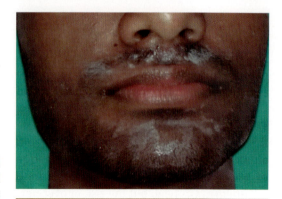

Figure 4: Pseudofrost with salicylic acid peel.

Photo courtesy: Dr Madan, Fellow of Cosmetic Dermatology, BMCRI

begins 2 days postpeel and can extend up to 7 days postpeel. The efficacy of salicylic acid peels is directly correlated to the degree of desquamation that is seen postpeel.[25] Bland cleansers and moisturizers are continued for 48 hours or until all postpeel irritation subsides.

Side Effects

- Transient hyperpigmentation and superficial crusting may be seen in areas of inflammatory acne. Patients with Fitzpatrick skin type III may experience darkening during desquamation due to increased melanin sloughing (Figure 5)
- Rarely edema and transient purpura in the lower eyelid areas, hypopigmentation, transient dryness, and hyperpigmentation, which resolves quickly within 1–2 weeks. Transient ulcerations may occur when peels are attempted on nasolabial fold. (Figure 6)
- Salicylism has not been seen as a side effect postpeel since the total amount of SA applied is very small and the majority of the solution is removed once the solution has volatized.

Trichloroacetic Acid

Trichloroacetic acid (TCA) occurs naturally as a colorless crystal and is easily

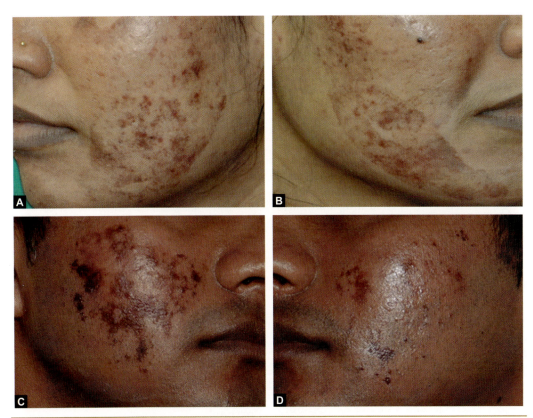

Figure 5: Rag burns caused due to salicylic acid peel. **A** and **B**, Burn appearance day after peel. Recovery is complete. **C** and **D**, Burn response can be unpredictable as cheeks of this patient shows.

Photo Courtesy: Derma-Care, Mangaluru.

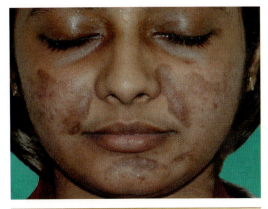

Figure 6: Peels should not be attempted in nasolabial fold as it can lead to ulceration. Patient underwent salicylic peel. Healing is prolonged but complete.

Photo Courtesy: Derma-Care, Mangaluru.

formulated by mixture with distilled water. Trichloroacetic acid is stable under normal conditions with a melting point of 54°C. It is not light sensitive; however, it is hygroscopic, so the crystals should be stored in a closed container to limit its absorption of water. Once mixed, TCA has a shelf life of at least 2 years. Selection of appropriate strength TCA is critical when performing a peel. The use of TCA in strengths greater than 35% should be discouraged with the exception of deliberate destruction of isolated lesions or where intentional controlled scarring is desired such as the treatment of ice-pick scars.[26] As a rule, nonfacial skin takes much longer to heal and is at much greater risk of scarring than when using a similar concentration on the face. This is due to the higher concentration of pilosebaceous units on the face compared with nonfacial sites.

Indications[26]

- Epidermal growths including actinic keratosis and thin seborrheic keratoses
- Mild to moderate photoaging
- Pigmentary dyschromias—melasma and postinflammatory hyperpigmentation
- Pigmented lesions including lentigines and ephelides
- Acne
- Acne scarring.

Procedure

A topical anesthetic such as 4% lidocaine may be used prior to application of the TCA to reduce patient discomfort with burning and stinging. Routine procedure of application is followed. The endpoint of peel is frosting (Figure 7).

Classification

Classification of TCA is given in table 4.

Once the desired frost is achieved, the skin can be rinsed off with water, or cooled down with cool wet compresses which are applied to the skin.

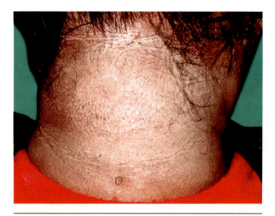

Figure 7: Frosting with trichloroacetic acid peel.

TABLE 4: The following classification can be used as a general guideline for trichloroacetic acid peels	
Level 1	Erythema with blotchy or wispy areas of white frosting. This indicates a superficial epidermal peel as can be achieved with trichloroacetic acid concentrations <30%; this peel will result in light flaking lasting 2–4 days
Level 2	White frosting with areas of erythema showing through. This level of peel is indicative of a full-thickness epidermal and can be achieved with trichloroacetic acid concentration of >30%; this peel will result in full exfoliation of the epidermis
Level 3	Solid white frosting with no erythema. This is indicative of penetration of trichloroacetic acid through the papillary dermis and can also be achieved with trichloroacetic acid concentrations >30%, depending on the number of applications

Postpeel

With superficial TCA peels, there may be mild-to-moderate erythema with fine flaking of the skin, lasting up to 4 days. With medium-depth TCA peels, patients should be advised that the peeled skin will feel and look tight. Pre-existing pigmented lesions will darken considerably, and appear grayish to brown. There is also a varying degree of erythema and edema. Edema may last several days (peaks at 48 h) and patients should elevate their head while sleeping. Frank desquamation typically begins by the third day and is accompanied by serous exudation. Re-epithelialization is usually complete by the 7th to 10th day. Although superficial TCA peels can be repeated every 4–6 weeks, medium-depth chemical peels should not be repeated for a period of 6 months, until the phases of healing are completed.

Side Affects

- Postinflammatory hyperpigmentation
- Prolonged erythema—localized areas of prolonged erythema, particularly on the angle of the jaw can be indicative of incipient scarring
- With deep peels, there are risks of infections (bacterial, viral, fungal), milia, acne, textural changes, and scarring. Milia formation is most likely due to over occlusion and can be minimized with the use of less occlusive emollients after re-epithelialization.

Pyruvic Acid

Pyruvic acid is α-keto-acid, and has been recently used as a medium chemical peeling agent in concentrations of 40–70%. It converts physiologically into lactic acid.

Indications[27]

- Inflammatory acne
- Moderate acne scars
- Greasy skin
- Actinic keratosis
- Warts
- Melasma.

Procedure

Apply the solution to small areas (forehead, one cheek at a time, chin, nose, and upper lip) and neutralize each area with sodium bicarbonate before progressing to the next area. A small fan should be used during the application of pyruvic acid to avoid inhaling the vapors.[28] Endpoint is the appearance of erythema. Pyruvic acid is then inactivated by the application of a solution of 10% sodium bicarbonate in water. Treatments can be repeated every 2 weeks for a total of 1–3 months.[29]

Postpeel

Mild erythema generally persists for a few hours after peeling which is followed by a very mild desquamation, persisting for 7–10 days after peeling.

Retinoic Acid Peel

Retinoic acid peels are also known as yellow peels, in which the concentration of peeling agent is 5–10%.

Indications

- Facial melanosis
- Axillary pigmentation
- Acne
- Photoaging.[30]

Specific Contraindications

- Rosacea
- Telangiectasia.

Procedure

Two to three coats of peeling agent are applied till a uniform yellow frost is seen and patient is sent home. They are instructed to wash off the peel after 4 hours. Procedure can be repeated every 15 days.

Side Effects

As it is a very superficial peel, not many side effects are reported.

Jessner's Solution

Jessner's peel is a solution that combines resorcinol (14 g), salicylic acid (14 g), 85% lactic acid (14 g), and 95% ethanol to make a solution of 100 mL. Jessner's solution was formulated to lower the concentration and toxicity of any one agent and to enhance the keratolytic effects.

Indications

- Inflammatory and comedonal acne
- Melasma
- Hyperkeratotic skin disorders
- Postinflammatory hyperpigmentation
- Lentigines
- Freckles
- Photodamage.

Contraindications

Allergies to resorcinol, salicylic acid, or lactic acid are absolute contraindications.

Procedure

Jessner's solution is applied to the skin with 2" × 2" gauze or a sable brush, which produces erythema and a very light frost within 15–45 seconds. The clinical endpoint of treatment is the erythema and blotchy frosting. The depth of penetration of the peeling agent is related to the number of coats applied. For superficial peeling, two coats are usually applied. Additional coats increase the depth of peeling. The advantages of Jessner's solution are that only a single solution is needed, timing the duration of application is unnecessary, and dilution or "neutralization" is not performed.

Side Effects

- Increased exfoliation in some patients
- Though there are concerns regarding resorcinol toxicity, including thyroid dysfunction risk assessment, studies have shown that under real-life conditions, human exposures to resorcinol are not expected to cause adverse effects on thyroid function.[28]

Combinations

Jessner's peel can also be combined with 5-fluorouracil delivered in a weekly pulse dose regimen, also known as the fluor-hydroxy

TABLE 5: Results of peels with type of lesions	
Good results	Variable to poor results
Very superficial, superficial, and medium depth peels	
• Freckles • Epidermal melasma • Superficial wrinkles • Acne • Seborrhea • Photoaging—grade 1 and 2	• Lentigenes • Dermal and mixed melasma • Proliferative lesions like seborrheic keratosis
Deep peels	
• Freckles • Lentigenes • Small seborrheic keratosis • Advanced photoaging	• Nevi • Dermal melasma

pulse peel, to treat actinic keratosis with an associated improvement in cosmesis.

Modified Jessner's—17% lactic acid, 17% salicylic acid, 8% citric acid, and ethanol (sufficient quantity to make 100 mL).

Table 5 lists the result of the peel with type of lesions.

❏ CONCLUSION

For a safe and effective practice with chemical peels, select appropriate patient, spend adequate time on counseling, and take informed written consent. Know about the chemical agent which is being used well. Priming the patient before procedure gives enhanced results and reduces many side effects. It is preferable to do a test peel, especially if a new agent is used. Do not leave the room to attend other chores when a procedure is being done. For timed peels, watch for erythema or severe burning to neutralize the peel. Postpeel photoprotection and possible side effects should be explained.

❏ REFERENCES

1. Khunger N. Standard guidelines of care for chemical peels. Indian J Dermatol Venereol Leprol. 2008;74:S5-12.

2. Stephen W. Perkins. Chemical peel. In: Cummings CW, editor. Otolaryngology-head and neck surgery. Maryland Heights: Mosby Publication; 1998. p. 640.

3. Kligman D, Kligman AM. Salicylic acid peels for the treatment of photoaging. Dermatol Surg. 1998;24:325-8.

4. Chemical peels. In: Rubin MG, editor. Procedures in cosmetic dermatology. Philadelphia: Elsevier Inc.; 2006. p. 1-12.

5. Khunger N. Step by step chemical peels. New Delhi: Jaypee Brothers Medical Publishers (P) Ltd.; 2010. p. 20.

6. Rubin ME. Superficial and medium depth. In: Manual of chemical peels. Philadelphia: Lippincott; 1995. p. 17-25.

7. Garg VK, Sarkar R, Agarwal R. Comparative evaluation of beneficiary effects of priming agents (2% hydroquinone and 0.025% retinoic acid) in the treatment of melasma with glycolic acid peels. Dermatol Surg. 2008;34(8):1032-9; discussion 1340.

8. Swinehart JM. Test spots in dermabrasion and chemical peeling. J Dermatol Surg Oncol 16:557-63.

9. Ditre CM. Glycolic acid peels. Dermatol Ther. 2000;13(2):165-72.

10. Fabbrocini G, De Padova MPD, Tosti A. Chemical peels: what's new and what isn't new but still works well. Facial Plast Surg. 2009;25(5):329-36.

11. Khunger N. Step by step chemical peels. New Delhi: Jaypee Brothers Medical Publishers (P) Ltd.; 2010. p. 69.

12. Landau M. Chemical peels. Clin Dermatol. 2008;26(2):200-8.

13. Sharad J. Glycolic acid peel therapy—a current review. Clin Cosmet Investig Dermatol. 2013;6:281-8.

14. Khunger N, Taneja D, Khunger M. Glycolic acid peels. In: Mysore V, (Ed). ACSI Textbook on cutaneous and aesthetic surgery. New Delhi: Jaypee Brothers Medical Publishers (P) Ltd.; 2012. p. 584.

15. Nikalji N, Godse K, Sakhiya J, Patil S, Nadkarni N. Complications of medium depth and deep chemical peels. J Cutaneous Aesthet Surg. 2012;5(4):254-60.

16. Moy LS. Superficial chemical peels with alpha-hydroxy acids. In: Robinson JK, Arndt KA, Le Boit PE, Wintroub BU, (Eds). Atlas of cutaneous surgery. Philadelphia: WB Saunders; 1996. pp. 345-50.

17. Marrero GM, Katz BE. The new fluor-hydroxy pulse peel. A combination of 5-fluorouracil and glycolic acid. Dermatol Surg. 1998;24(9):973-8.

18. Rendon MI, Effron C, Edison BL. The use of fillers and botulinum toxin type A in combination with superficial glycolic acid (alpha-hydroxy acid) peels: optimizing injection therapy with the skin-smoothing properties of peels. Cutis. 2007;79(1 Suppl Combining):9-12.

19. Sharquie KE, Al-Tikreety MM, Al-Mashhadani SA. Lactic acid as a new therapeutic peeling agent in melasma. Dermatol Surg. 2005;31(2):149-54.

20. Sharquie KE, Al-Tikreety MM, Al-Mashhadani SA. Lactic acid chemical peels as a new therapeutic modality in melasma in comparison to Jessner's solution chemical peels. Dermatol Surg. 2006;32(12):1429-36.

21. Lee HS, Kim IH. Salicylic acid peels for the treatment of acne vulgaris in Asian patients. Dermatol Surg. 2003;29:1196-9.

22. James PE, Salicylic acid. In: Tosti A, Grimes PA, Padova MPD, (Eds). Color atlas of chemical peels. Berlin Heidelberg: Springer; 2012. p. 51.

23. Vedamurthy M. Salicylic acid peels. Indian J Dermatol Venereol Leprol. 2004;70:136-8.

24. Khunger N. Chemical peel. In: Valia RG, Valia AR, (Eds). IADVL Textbook of Dermatology. 3rd ed. Mumbai: Bhalani Publishing House; 2008. p. 1678-87.

25. Grimes PE. Salicylic acid. In: Tosti A, Grimes PA, Padova MPD, editors. Color Atlas of Chemical Peels. Berlin Heidelberg: Springer; 2012. pp. 55.

26. Harmon CB, Hadley M, Tristani P. Trichloroacetic acid. In: Tosti A, Grimes PA, Padova MPD, (Eds). Color atlas of chemical peels. Berlin Heidelberg: Springer; 2012.pp. 61-4.

27. Berardesca E, Cameli N, Primavera G, Carrera M. Clinical and instrumental evaluation of skin improvement after treatment with a new 50% pyruvic acid peel. Dermatol Surg. 2006;32(4):526-31.

28. Tosti A, Grimes PA, Padova MPD, (Eds). Color atlas of chemical peels. Berlin Heidelberg: Springer; 2012. pp.31-8.

29. Tosson Z, Attwa E, Al-Mokadem S. Pyruvic acid as a new therapeutic peeling agent in acne, melasma and warts. Egyptian Dermatology Online Journal. 2006;2(2).

30. Sharad J. Newer chemical peels. In: Mysore V, (Eds). ACSI textbook on cutaneous and aesthetic surgery. New Delhi: Jaypee Brothers Medical Publishers (P) Ltd.; 2012. p. 595.

Excimer Lasers: Optimizing Results and Minimizing Complications

Sanjeev J Aurangabadkar, Sanjay Dubey

❏ INTRODUCTION

Lasers have become an integral part of dermatology practice. Their applications encompass cosmetic indications, such as rejuvenation, hair reduction, and tattoo removal on the one hand and therapeutic indications, such as for the management of vitiligo and psoriasis on the other. Often, these lasers yield gratifying results but are limited by their availability, the cost involved, prolonged treatment duration, etc. Despite the evolution in technology and techniques, complications do occur and dermatologists have to be geared up to face these challenges. The choice of equipment, protocol, and patient selection also play a major role in the predictability of adverse effects. This chapter outlines the rational use of 308 nm excimer laser, its complications, and their management. Vitiligo carries immense social stigma and causes significant psycosocial distress in patients and this chapter primarily focuses on excimer laser in this condition.[1]

An excimer laser device uses a combination of a noble gas (such as xenon) and a reactive gas (such as chlorine), which upon proper electrical stimulation and under pressure, produces an excimer pseudomolecule (Figure 1). This molecule exists in an energized state and releases photons in the ultraviolet spectrum, and more specifically a wavelength of 308 nm ultraviolet (UV) light.[2-4]

Narrow band UV B (NBUVB) phototherapy is an established modality to treat vitiligo and psoriasis. Narrow band UV B has immunomodulating effects and also can stimulate the melanocytes in the outer root sheaths (ORS) of hair follicles. The 308 nm excimer laser produces photobiological effects similar to NBUVB.[5]

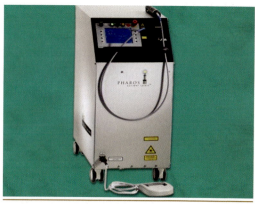

Figure 1: Excimer laser system.

These include:

- Direct cytotoxic effects on infiltrating T cells in the skin
- T cell apoptosis
- Stimulation of melanocytes proliferation and migration from reservoirs in the hair follicles.

This forms the basis of the postulated mechanism of action of excimer lasers. The advantage of these devices over NBVUB include more rapid repigmentation response, selective treatment of affected areas, thus sparing UV exposure to uninvolved skin, and safety in children.

❑ INDICATIONS

- Vitiligo[4]
- Psoriasis[5]
- Hypopigmented striae distensae and hypopigmented scars.[6]

❑ PATIENT SELECTION: WHICH TO AVOID AND WHY

Proper patient selection is important prior to starting excimer laser therapy. As a general rule, patients with darker skin tones respond better to this treatment.

Patients with unstable vitiligo are best avoided and those with lesions on the face and upper trunk respond better to therapy than those on acral areas.[7] As treatments are performed at weekly or biweekly intervals, the patient needs to have high motivation to undergo therapy and involves significant time commitment.[8]

It is important to avoid patients with unrealistic expectations (they need to be aware that the purpose of treatment is repigmentation and not cure).

Increased frequency with lesions on UV resistant area such as elbows, knees, wrists, ankles, and dorsa of hands and feet as the response generally poor.[7] In the authors experience, these are areas where one would use laser and targeted phototherapy the most since these are resistant areas and need higher joules.

It is prudent to avoid photosensitive patients such as those with conditions like:

- Systemic lupus erythematosus
- Discoid lupus erythematosus
- Dermatitis pigmentosa
- Porphyria
- Actinic dermatosis.
- It is also logical to avoid patients with the following:
- Past excessive actinic exposure
- Patients with any injury or infection over the lesion
- Patients with history of seizures.

❑ LASER TECHNIQUE AND PROTOCOL

Excimer lasers have a hand piece with a fixed spot size covering a large area (square or a round spot) (Figure 2). In order to treat a smaller lesion or of varying shapes and sizes, customized stencils can be used to treat a given lesion to match it and avoid undue exposure

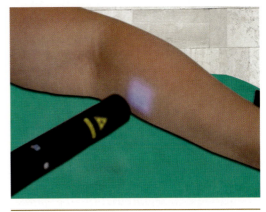

Figure 2: Excimer laser handpiece depicting spot size.

to surrounding areas. The handpiece is held perpendicular to the skin and laser shots fired with a foot switch. Treatments are performed once or twice weekly till repigmentation is achieved. Average number of sessions tend to be 20–30 in number.[9,10]

- Patients selection: this is the singlemost important criterion for successful outcome and reducing complication risk. The patient needs to be in stable state, as laser given in active stage may lead to koebnerization
- Maximum area to be taken for laser should be only up to 6–7 % of body area (in authors personal experience)
- Since it is a collimated light, avoid the overlapping while doing the procedure
- Take all safety precautions which include protecting glasses too
- Explain every possible complication and always take a written consent form and pre- and postprocedure photographs
- Dose on site, e.g., acral sites need higher doses and sensitive areas like lips, nipple, vagina, glans penis, and perianal areas need lower doses
- The resulting erythema may help to decide the dose titration
- No anesthesia is generally necessary
- Unaffected skin is covered by stencils or UV protecting templates to minimize exposure of uninvolved skin
- Perform minimal erythema dose (MED) testing if necessary. The minimal dose that produces confluent erythema within 24 hours is called MED
- Start with MED dose and then increase dose by about $50 \, mJ/cm^2$ every subsequent session to produce erythema. This is very subjective as patients sensitivity may vary[11]
- Multiple sessions are necessary to achieve satisfactory regimentation. Response depends upon more on total number of sessions and frequency of sessions.[12]

❑ COMPLICATIONS AND THEIR MANAGEMENT

As with any laser therapy, risks of adverse effects always exist. Most of these tend to be transient and self-limiting. Permanent sequels such as scarring have not been reported with excimer laser.[13-15] Proper patient selection and adherence to protocol is the key to avoid untoward events. Most of these are technique dependant. It is important to avoid overlapping while treating large contiguous areas and gradual increments in dose is preferred.

Some of the complications are listed below:

- Pruritus
- Koebnerization
- Hypererythema
- Burns
- Dyschromias and hyperpigmentation
- Blistering
- Xerosis and scaling
- Ecchymoses and petichiae.

Some of these are discussed below with tips on how to manage them.

Koebnerization

Koebner phenomenon or isomorphic phenomenon where new lesions appear on sites of trauma or injury is known to occur in vitiligo (Figure 3). Treating unstable cases carries this risk where laser therapy may induce new lesions when excess dose is used. Laser or targeted phototherapy in active disease should not be used as it may worsen the lesions. It is advisable to treat stable vitiligo as shown in figure 3.

Hypererythema

Erythema is a desirable endpoint with excimer lasers (Figure 4). On use of appropriate energy/fluence, erythema can be anticipated and this is followed by repigmentation. However, in some instances, even in stable vitiligo and

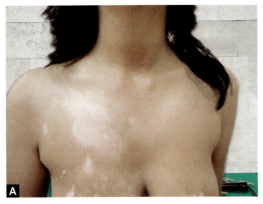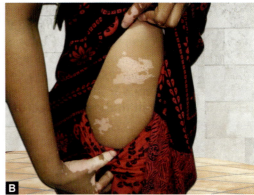

Figure 3: Koebnerization.

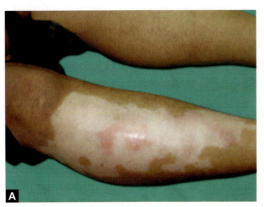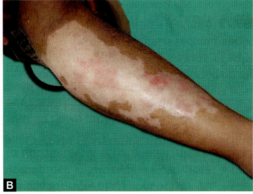

Figure 4: Erythema following excimer laser treatment.

where prior doses did not produce erythema or burning, patients may abruptly develop excessive erythema and skin may become hypersensitive on dose increments. This possibility needs to be explained to the patients before commencing the procedure. The best way to avoid this is follow slow increments in dose.

Hyperpigmentation

This can be seen often on treated areas and surrounding rim of lesions, and can be avoided by reducing doses and reduce frequency of therapy, although in Indian patients,

erythema and hyperpigmentation gives a positive psychological impact (Figure 5). The use of proper stencils and matching the spot size of the laser to the lesion will minimize perilesional hyperpigmentation. The patient also needs to avoid excess sun exposure to the treated area as this may also cause hyper pigmentation.

Tip

To avoid hyper pigmentation, reduce dose and frequency (the authors usually space sessions once a week) and use topical steroids for short duration.

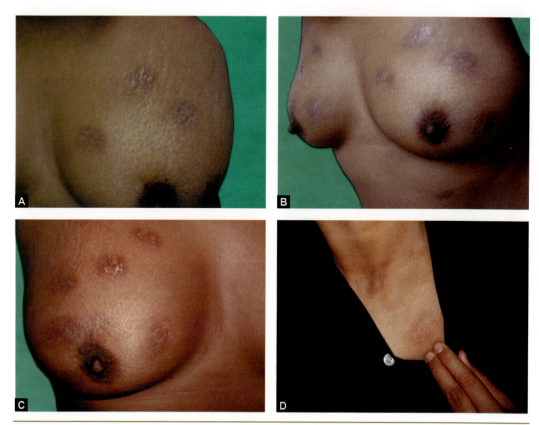

Figure 5: Hyperpigmentation following excimer laser therapy.

Dyschromasia

Patchy or uneven repigmentation can occur during therapy (Figure 6).

Tip

This is best handled by stopping treatment and letting the skin distribute melanin (full body phototherapy can be continued during this time).

Xerosis

Dryness and scaling or exfoliation (like in cases of sun burn) can occur after excimer laser therapy (Figure 7).

Tip

Using emollients and moisturizers usually suffices to overcome this.

Burn

This usually occurs on use of excessive energy following excimer laser therapy (Figure 8). This can be avoided by lowering energy, gradual increments, and titration of dose according to skin types and MED testing.

Ecchymosis and Petechiae

This is a rare complication which the authors have come across (Figure 9).

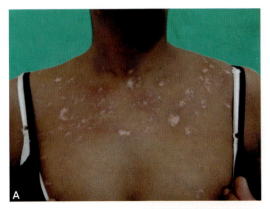
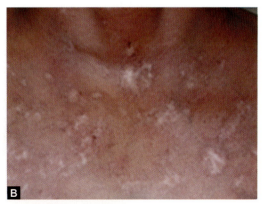
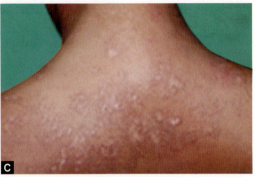

Figure 6: Dyschromia following excimer laser.

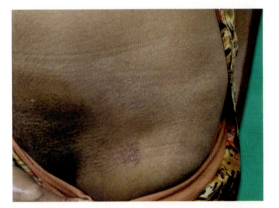

Figure 7: Xerosis and scaling following excimer laser therapy.

Blisters

If blistering occurs, stop treatment and give topical and oral anti-inflammatory along with good counseling. Blistering is best managed by advising the patient to use antibiotic or petrolatum ointment topically (Figure 10).

❏ CONCLUSION

Excimer lasers have an established role to play in the management of vitiligo. It offers the fastest repigmentation with least number of sessions compared to conventional phototherapy and is safe to perform even in children and in pregnancy. Though the therapy is remarkably safe, complications do occur and these can be minimized by following proper protocols and careful patient selection. Complications tend to be easily manageable with no permanent sequel. The therapy can be extremely gratifying for both the patient and

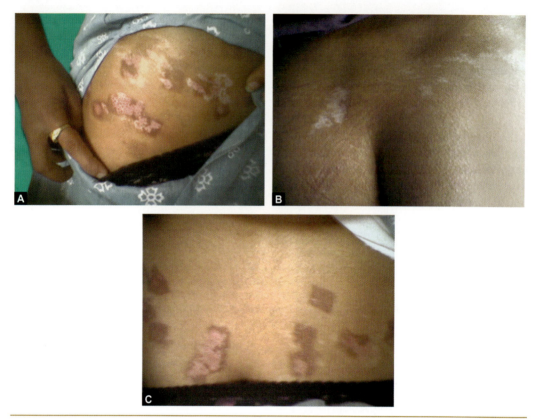

Figure 8: Burns following excimer laser.

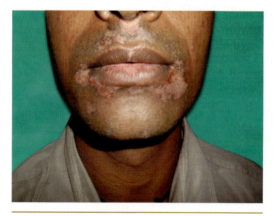

Figure 9: Petechiae after excimer.

physician alike. To conclude, complications can be managed but excimer lasers are very expensive and not practical in Indian scenario because of its high cost and less benefit if we compare with other modalities like targeted phototherapy.

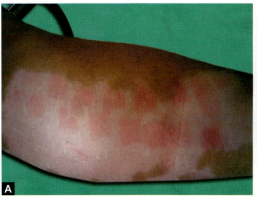 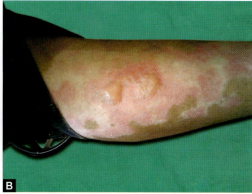

Figure 10: Blistering following excimer laser therapy.

❑ REFERENCES

1. Ongenae K, Beelaert L, van Geel N, Naeyaert JM. Psychosocial effects of vitiligo. J Eur Acad Dermatol Venereol. 2006;20:1-8.

2. Spencer JM, Hadi SM. The excimer lasers. J Drugs Dermatol. 2004;3:522-5.

3. Repigmentation of localized vitiligo with the xenon chloride laser. Br J Dermatol. 2001;144:1266-7.

4. Spencer JM, Nossa R, Ajmeri J. Treatment of vitiligo with the 308-nm excimer laser: a pilot study. J Am Acad Dermatol. 2002;46:727-31.

5. Feldman SR, Mellen BG, Housman TS, Fitzpatrick RE, Geronemus RG, Friedman PM, et al. Efficacy of 308-nm excimer laser for treatment of psoriasis: results of a multi-center study. J Am Acad Dermatol. 2002;46(6):900-6.

6. Baltas E, Nagy P, Bonis B, Novak Z, Ignacz F, Szabo G, et al. Sarradet D, Hussein M, Solana LG, Goldberg DJ (2002) Repigmentation of striae with a 308nm excimer laser. Lasers Med Surg 14(Suppl):44-45

7. Hofer A, Hassan AS, Legat FJ, Kerl H, Wolf P. The efficacy of excimer laser (308 nm) for vitiligo at different body sites. J Eur Acad Dermatol Venereol. 2006;20:558-64.

8. Hofer A, Hassan AS, Legat FJ, Kerl H, Wolf P. Optimal weekly frequency of 308-nm excimer laser treatment in vitiligo patients. Br J Dermatol. 2005;152:981-5.

9. Hadi S, Tinio P, Al-Ghaithi K, Al-Qari H, Al-Helalat M, Lebwohl, M, et al. Treatment of vitiligo using the 308-nm excimer laser. Photomed Laser Surg. 2006;24:354-7.

10. Passeron T, Ortonne JP. Use of the 308-nm excimer laser for psoriasis and vitiligo. Clin Dermatol. 2006;24:33-42.

11. Choi KH, Park JH, Ro YS. Treatment of vitiligo with 308-nm xenon-chloride excimer laser: therapeutic efficacy of different initial doses according to treatment areas. J Dermatol. 2004;31:284-92.

12. Ostovari N, Passeron T, Zakaria W, Fontas E, Larouy JC, Blot JF, et al. Treatment of vitiligo by 308-nm excimer laser: an evaluation of variables affecting treatment response. Lasers Surg Med. 2004;35:152-6.

13. Majid I. Efficacy of targeted narrowband ultraviolet B therapy in Vitiligo. Indian J Dermatol 2014;59:485-9

14. Kanwar AJ, Kumaran M S. Childhood vitiligo: treatment paradigms. Indian J Dermatol. 2012;57:466-74.

15. Asawanonda P, Anderson R, Chang Y, Taylor CR. 308-nm excimer laser for the treatment of psoriasis: A dose-response study. Arch Dermatol. 2000;136(5):619-24.

Adverse Effects of Dermabrasion and Microdermabrasion

Anil Ganjoo, Shikhar Ganjoo

❑ HISTORICAL BACKGROUND AND EVOLUTION OF TECHNIQUE

Aged skin is characterized by epidermal and dermal atrophy, presence of wrinkles, irregular pigmentation, telangiectasia, and flaccidity. With increasing technological advances, there are many options for cosmetic procedures that minimize skin changes associated with aging. Among them are dermabrasion and microdermabrasion. The history of dermabrasion dates back to 16th century Egypt, but its introduction in the plastic surgery literature occurred in 1947, when Iverson described a technique of planing skin to the dermis with sandpaper in order to correct traumatic tattoos.[1] The technique was further refined by Kurtin in 1953, who pioneered the use of the mechanized wire brush, specifically for acne scars. For the past 50 years, dermabrasion has also been used to improve surgical and traumatic scars. In 1988, Yarborough found in an observational study that dermabrasion with a wire brush performed 4–8 weeks after the initial injury achieved excellent correction, changing the widely held impression that scars had to be treated at a greater interval after injury.[2,3]

As a means of planing surgical surfaces and improving photodamaged skin, dermabrasion has been compared with laser resurfacing and different methods of dermabrasion have been developed. Applying the technique with sterile sandpaper (sometimes referred to as dermasanding) was shown to be equivalent to dermabrasion with the motor-powered diamond fraise. The term "electrobrasion" is used to represent a distinct means of surgical planing using the common office electrosurgical unit. Electrosurgical resurfacing has been described at least as far back as 1999. Earlier observations that precise ablation could be achieved by adjusting power settings and tissue contact time prompted the question of how the technique of electrobrasion worked compared with traditional dermabrasion. The observed benefits of electrosurgical resurfacing techniques include ease of use and decreased cost of equipment, relative to laser ablation.[4]

❑ INTRODUCTION

Microdermabrasion consists of negative-pressure systems, which pass aluminum oxide crystals onto the skin, while simultaneously vacuuming the used crystals. Microdermabrasion treatment promoted skin rejuvenation through an increase in skin thickness due to an increase in epidermal thickness and collagen organization. This treatment causes little or no bleeding, and fewer complications. There is no need for local anesthesia or high surgical skills compared with traditional dermabrasion.[5,6]

However, in the authors' experience, if the operator is not careful and uniform in movement, there may be superficial abrasions that may end up with pigmentory disturbances or superficial scarring. So it is imperative to be gentle and uniform while doing the procedure and also to apply gentle vacuum to start with and then build up the pressure gradually.

❑ CURRENT LITERATURE ON COMPLICATIONS AND AUTHOR'S EXPERIENCE

Farris and Rietschel[7] did a study to determine if latex exposure caused an acute urticarial response following microdermabrasion in a latex-allergic patient. The patient was prick tested to saline and histamine controls, latex, and sterile medical grade 100 m aluminum oxide crystals that had been passed through the microdermabrader. The strongly positive latex prick test confirmed latex allergy in the patient. Negative prick testing to aluminum oxide crystals that had passed through the microdermabrader make it unlikely that the patient was exposed to latex via this system. Physicians need to carefully evaluate patients who are considering microdermabrasion and appreciate that unexpected serious complications can occur.

Dermabrasion has many potential complications, most of which are often operator and technique dependent. Photosensitivity occurs universally postprocedure, and patients must use strict sun protection while the skin re-epithelializes. Additionally, erythema after dermabrasion can last several weeks to months, and can be treated in part with topical corticosteroids. Postinflammatory pigmentation alterations, especially hypopigmentation, are frequent complications that can be permanent. Postprocedural hypertrophic scarring is a potential risk. This phenomenon was first reported in patients undergoing dermabrasion after receiving a recent course of isotretinoin therapy. As a result, it is currently recommended that patients wait at least 6 months after completion of isotretinoin therapy before undergoing a dermabrasion procedure. Despite this recommendation, there are reports of patients undergoing dermabrasion with current isotretinoin therapy, without hypertrophic scar formation.[8,9]

The authors recommend that the patients should be primed with a triple combination or hydroquinone or retinoids at least 2 weeks prior to the dermabrasion sessions. Also strict sun protection should be prescribed between the sessions and thereafter. This can go a long way to prevent complications like postprocedure hyperpigmentation and hypopigmentation.

Gogia and Grekin[10] reported eruptive self-resolving keratoacanthomas that developed after treatment with photodynamic therapy and microdermabrasion. Microdermabrasion is well tolerated by most patients and minimal side effects have been reported, among which are a mild to moderate erythema, which lasts on average 1 or 2 days after treatment, mild discomfort during the procedure, and a tingling sensation. Literature describes only uncomfortable feeling of a low intensity that occurred during the procedure and the appearance of mild to moderate erythema after the procedure lasting up to 2 days. The negative pressure applied to the skin is also responsible for the appearance of erythema, partly by increasing local blood circulation, and may contribute to faster healing and repair.[11]

In the authors practice, mild erythema persisting for a few weeks after the procedure has been experienced. This is usually self-limiting and resolves on its own. Resolution may be hastened with use of emollients containing hyaluronic acid that maintains moisture and suppleness of the skin. Of course sun protection has to be strictly followed to avoid development of postinflammatory hyperpigmentation.

Svider and Jiron[12] did a study to enumerate the factors raised in litigation following these procedures that included poor cosmetic outcome (80%), alleged intratreatment negligence (68%), permanent injury (64%), informed-consent deficits (60%), emotional/psychological injury (44%), post-treatment negligence (32%), and the need for additional treatment/surgery (32%).

Kim and Lim[13] did a study with an objective to see changes in transepidermal water loss (TEWL), hydration, and erythema of the face following diamond microdermabrasion. Twenty-eight patients were included in this spilt face study. Transepidermal water loss, stratum corneum hydration, and the degree of erythema were measured from the right and left sides of the face (forehead and cheek) at baseline. One side of the face was treated with diamond microdermabrasion and the other side was left untreated. Measurements were taken right after the procedure and repeated at set time intervals. Diamond microdermabrasion was associated with a statistically significant increase in TEWL immediately after the procedure and at 24 hours. However, on day 2, levels of TEWL were back to baseline. An increase in hydration and erythema was observed right after microdermabrasion, but both returned to baseline on day 1. The results of their study showed that skin barrier function of the forehead and cheek recovers within 2 days of diamond microdermabrasion. Diamond microdermabrasion performed on a weekly basis, as presently done, is expected to allow sufficient time for the damaged skin to recover its barrier function in most parts of the face.

The authors recommend that the skin of every patient be assessed before each session and factors like skin hydration, turgor, and texture should be taken into account. If the skin is dry or irritated, the procedure can be postponed until the skin becomes better. This will prevent the development of side effects. Also maintenance of hydration of the skin postdermabrasion is extremely important since the deficient epidermis during the postprocedure period is prone to TEWL and dehydration. So hyaluronic acid based moisturizers are of great help.

Fakhouri and Harmon[14] reported a very serious side effect in which the patient developed subarachnoid hemorrhage during dermabrasion for scar revision and was on of direct thrombin inhibitors.

Local side effects are uncommon and transient but include pain, burning, sensitive skin, photosensitivity, tiger stripes, or diffuse hyperpigmentation. Workers who routinely inhale silica dust (silicosis), asbestos fibers (asbestosis), or hard metal dust are at risk of pulmonary fibrosis. Hence, the operator must protect himself/herself with a mask. The crystals may also get into the eyes of the operator or more commonly the patient. Hence, the patient must wear protective eyewear during the procedure.[15]

❑ CONCLUSION

To conclude, both dermabrasion and micro-dermabrasion are popular nonsurgical skin resurfacing techniques which are relatively safe in experienced hands. A proper patient assessment prior to both the procedures and maintenance of hydration postprocedure can further minimize the already low complication rate.

❑ REFERENCES

1. Lawrence N, Mandy S, Yarborough J, Alt T. History of dermabrasion. Dermatol Surg. 2000;26:95-101.
2. Iverson PC. Surgical removal of traumatic tattoos of the face. Plast Reconstr Surg. 1946;1947:427-32.
3. Robbins N. Dr Abner Kurtin, father of ambulatory dermabrasion. J Dermatol Surg Oncol. 1988;14:425-31.
4. Kleinerman R, Armstrong AW, Ibrahimi OA, King TH, Eisen DB. Electrobrasion vs. manual dermabrasion: a randomized, double-blind, comparative effectiveness trial. British J Dermatol. 2014;171:124-9.
5. Karimipour DJ, Kang S, Johnson TM, Orringer JS, Hamilton T, Hammerberg C, et al. Microdermabrasion with and without aluminum oxide crystal abrasion: a comparative molecular analysis of dermal remodelling. J Am Acad Dermatol. 2006;54:405-10.
6. Andrews SN, Zarnitsyn V, Bondy B, Prausnitz MR. Optimization of microdermabrasion for controlled removal of stratum corneum. Int J Pharm. 2011;407:95-104.
7. Farris PK, Rietschel RL. An unusual acute urticarial response following microdermabrasion. Dermtol Surg. 2002;28:606-8.
8. Fernandes M, Pinheiro NM, Crema VO, Mendonça AC. Effects of microdermabrasion on skin rejuvenation. J Cosmet Laser Ther. 2014;16:26-31
9. Kleinerman R, Armstrong AW, Ibrahimi OA, King TH, Eisen DB. Electrobrasion vs. manual dermabrasion: a randomized, double-blind, comparative effectiveness trial. Br J Dermatol. 2014;171:124-9.
10. Gogia R, Grekin RC, Shinkai K. Eruptive self-resolving keratoacanthomas developing after treatment with photodynamic therapy and microdermabrasion. Dermatol Surg. 2013;39:1717-20.
11. Fernandes M, Pinheiro NM, Crema VO, Mendonça AC. Effects of microdermabrasion on skin rejuvenation. J Cosmet Laser Ther. 2014;16:26-31.
12. Svider PF, Jiron J, Zuliani G, Shkoukani MA, Folbe AJ, Carron M. Unattractive Consequences: litigation from facial dermabrasion and chemical peels. Aesthet Surg J. 2014;34:1244-49.
13. Kim HS, Lim SH, Song JY, Kim MY, Lee JH, Park JG, et al. Skin barrier function recovery after diamond microdermabrasion. J Dermatol. 2009;36:529-33.
14. Fakhouri TM, Harmon CB. Hemorrhagic complications of direct thrombin inhibitors—subarachnoid hemorrhage during dermabrasion for scar revision. Dermatol Surg. 2013;39:1410 12.
15. Savardekar P. Microdermabrasion. Indian J Dermatol Venereol Leprol. 2007;73:277-9.

Platelet-rich Plasma

Kiran Godse, Aditya Mahajan

❑ INTRODUCTION

Platelet-rich plasma (PRP) (synonym: autologous platelet gel, plasma-rich growth factors, and platelet-concentrated plasma) means "abundant platelets that are concentrated into a small volume of plasma." There has been a growing interest in PRP as a procedure in dermatology in recent times. Its use has been studied in various indications from acne scars, facial rejuvenation, treatment of chronic scars, and various hair disorders.

❑ WHAT IS PLATELET-RICH PLASMA?

Platelets contain α-granules, which in turn contain various growth factors like transforming growth factor-β, platelet-derived growth factor, vascular endothelial growth factor, and fibroblasts. Degranulation growth factors in platelets occurs upon "activation". The secreted growth factors in turn bind to their respective transmembrane receptors expressed over adult mesenchymal stem cells, osteoblasts, fibroblasts, endothelial cells, and epidermal cells which induces an internal signal-transduction pathway, unlocking the expression of a normal gene sequence of a cell like cellular proliferation, matrix formation, osteoid production, collagen synthesis, etc., thereby augmenting the natural wound-healing process.[1]

Platelet-rich plasma has already attracted attention in plastic surgery, orthopedic surgery, and cardiac surgery because of its potential use in skin rejuvenating effects, rapid healing, reduced infection, and decreased chance of hypertrophic keloids and scars. Growth factors are known to activate the proliferative phase and transdifferentiation of hair and stem cells and produce new follicular units. Basic fibroblast growth factor is reported to promote the in vitro proliferation of papilla cells, and thereby plays a key role in elongating hair shaft.[2]

Many methods have been described for the isolation of PRP. The author uses the double spin manual method. The concentration obtained by the manual method was around 3–5 times the normal platelet concentration.

According to one study done by Khatu et al., the patient observed a significant reduction in hair loss between first and fourth injection.

They observed moderate improvement in hair coverage even on global photography. Overall, patient satisfaction was high with a mean result rating of 7.0 on a scale of 1–10 unsatisfactory results.

❑ INDICATIONS OF PLATELET-RICH PLASMA IN DERMATOLOGY[2]

- Androgenetic alopecia
- Alopecia areata
- Skin rejuvenation
- Acne scars and contour defects
- Wound ulcers, connective tissue disease associated ulcers
- Striae distensae
- Lipodermatosclerosis
- Lichen sclerosus.

❑ PROCEDURE

The method of isolating PRP are as follows:
- Collect 12 cc of blood in a blue topped Vacutainer containing sodium citrate (Figure 1).
- The collected sample is then centrifuged at 2,000 rpm for 15 minutes (Figure 2)
- A buffy coat (red arrow), PRP (lower half of the upper portion), and a platelet-poor plasma (top half of the upper portion) zone is identified (Figure 3)
- The PRP along with buffy coat is separated into a plain bulb
- The separated PRP is recentrifuged @2,500 rpm for 5 minutes (Figure 4)
- The isolated PRP is activated by adding 10% calcium chloride (1:10 ratio) (Figure 5)
- After which it is immediately injected with an insulin syringe mainly in the distribution of the area affected by male pattern baldness
- It can be used with dermaroller, mesogun, or after fractional laser in skin rejuvenation.

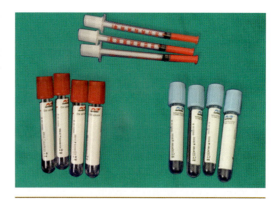

Figure 1: Blue topped (sodium citrate), red topped (plain) Vacutainers used for isolation of platelet-rich plasma.

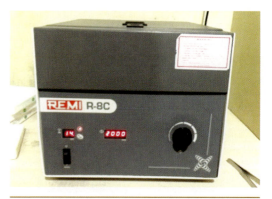

Figure 2: Remi R-8C® centrifuge being used to spin the isolated blood at 2,500 rpm for 10–15 minutes.

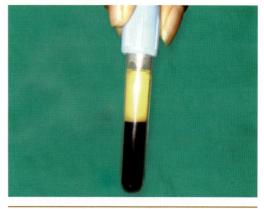

Figure 3: Identification of the "platelet poor" and the "platelet rich" zones.

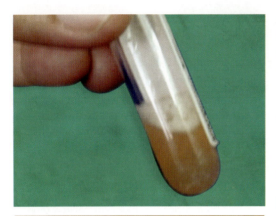

Figure 4: Isolated platelet-rich plasma.

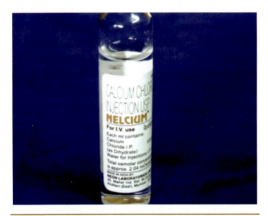

Figure 5: Injection calcium chloride Nelcium® added in 1:10 ratio.

Patient Preparation for Platelet-rich Plasma

Before the PRP applications, all patients were informed about the process and its potential adverse effects and should be asked to sign a consent form. They need not have their hair washed two days prior to the treatment. Local anesthesia (10% lignocaine spray, eutectic mixture of local anesthetics cream, or local block) was applied to the treatment area. Patient should be asked for history of medications (such as blood thinners, hypertensives, etc.). Any history of infectious disease like human

immunodeficiency virus (HIV), and hepatitis B surface antigen, hepatitis C virus should be ruled out. Pregnancy should also be ruled out. Sometimes it is advised prophylaxis with acyclovir or oral antibiotic in high risk cases.

Before the procedure, the patient should be asked to take a head bath with a routine shampoo and no oil application.

❑ COMPLICATIONS

Pain in the Injected Area, Headaches, and Heaviness of Head

Some people who have undergone PRP therapy complain about an acute ache or soreness in the spot of the injection. Sometimes this pain is even felt deep inside the area. This pain is transient and goes away with time. Topical anesthetic sprays or ice pack use can reduce it.

Swelling and Redness

There is common occurrence of mild, transient swelling over the area of injection. It can be due to the multiple injections causing mild inflammatory reaction. But it is not a serious complication and a transient one, which can be reduced postprocedural with ice-packs. This can also be due to the anesthesia.

Infection

Sometimes an infection can break out in the injured area. It can be viral or bacterial. Treatment is with routine antivirals and antibacterials. Pretreatment prophylaxis can also be considered.

No Improvement in Injured Area

While this is not necessarily a side-effect, we still need to mention that not all patients will respond to PRP. It is necessary to insist that PRP is an adjuvant therapy and not mainstay.

Allergic Reactions

Urticarial rash can occur after PRP Injection which can be treated with antihistamines.

Skin Discoloration

Sometimes the color around the skin of a PRP injection will appear bruised. This is very rare. Blood mixed PRP may give rise to pigmentation due to hemosiderin.

Bleeding

Patients with bleeding tendency or those who are on blood thinners can complain of bleeding. For this, proper history and advising the patient to stop blood thinners can be done. Transient bleeding is observed even in normal patients also, rarely it is a cause of concern for the clinician. Growth factors might have the potential for tumorigenesis or promotion of atypia.

Production and activity of the body's endogenous growth factors are closely controlled by positive and negative feedback mechanisms.[3]

Cross Labeling of Samples

This can cause serious side effects like a severe hypersensitivity reaction which can be fatal. It can cause transmission of infections. Proper training of technician and labeling is the solution. Another idea is to take up one patient at a time and discard all left overs of the patient postprocedure. Use dedicated centrifuge for this procedure.[4]

Being an autologous preparation, PRP is devoid of any serious adverse effects, apart from local injection site reactions like pain or secondary infection, which can be avoided with proper precautions. PRP has no issues regarding transmission of infections such as hepatitis-B, C, or HIV.

❑ CONCLUSION

Platelet-rich plasma therapy is a new upcoming therapy in the treatment of various dermatological conditions. As it is an autologous transfer of platelets the risks of side effects are negligible. It can be used as an adjuvant to improve results along with proven modalities of treatment.

❑ REFERENCES

1. Arshdeep, Kumaran MS. Platelet-rich plasma in dermatology: Boon or a bane? Indian J Dermatol Venereol Leprol. 2014;80:5-14.
2. Khatu SS, More YE, Gokhale NR, Chavhan DC, Bendsure N. J Cutan Aesthet Surg. 2014;7(2):107-110.
3. Zemtsov A, Montalvo-Lugo V. Topically applied growth factors change skin cytoplasmic creatine kinase activity and distribution and produce abnormal keratinocyte differentiation in murine skin. Skin Res Technol. 2008; 14(3):370-5.
4. Godse K. Platelet rich plasma in androgenic alopecia: where do we stand? J Cutan Aesthet Surg. 2014;7:110-1.

Prevention of Ocular Complications

Harsha S Pai

❏ INTRODUCTION

Risk of eye injury and thus the need for eye protection is central to all laser operations. Beam hazards cause direct injury to the eye and non beam hazards such as plume cause high irritation. Every cosmetic laser procedure must constantly use eye protection for both patient and medical personnel.

❏ EYE CARE DURING LASERS

The laser lights can harm the eyes. Safety guidelines for the use of lasers for dermatologic purposes must be reviewed. The guidelines should ensure that protocols and procedures address the problem of assuring that appropriate laser eye protection is always chosen for the selected wavelength of the laser. Lasers should be clearly labelled as to their emitted wavelengths and type of laser. Further labeling should clearly indicate which wavelength is selected and in use. Laser eye protection should be clearly marked and indicate the wavelength and type of protection that is afforded as well as the optical density for the protection. Current laser eye protective technologies offer several wavelength protection. However, it is important to remember that all wavelengths will not be covered by a single laser eye protective goggle or shield.

Types of ocular injuries are wavelength specific. The degree of ocular damage is dependent on the laser irradiance, exposure time, and beam size. Lasers, such as carbon dioxide lasers which emit light in ultraviolet or infrared portion of the electromagnetic spectrum, are absorbed by the aqueous humor that is in the anterior segment of the eye. It damages the cornea and the crystalline lens as these structures have a high aqueous concentration.[1] Grade 1 (opalescence of the corneal epithelium) and grade 2 (epithelial loss) corneal damages are reversible, and grade 3 (corneal scarring with coagulation of substantia propria) are irreversible.[2] The lasers emitting energy in the visible portion of the electromagnetic spectrum penetrate deeper to the posterior segment of the eye, damaging the retina and choroid. The melanin and hemoglobin in the retina absorb the energy and leads to damage of the retina. Injury to the foveal region of the retina causes visual impairment.[3] The neodymium-doped yttrium aluminum garnet lasers, alexandrite lasers, and diode lasers can damage both the lens and the retina. The damage can occur by photoacoustic and thermal mechanisms.

Ocular injury can occur from direct or indirect exposure. Injury to the eye can also occur from light scattered off the reflective surfaces such as glass, polished metal, or plastic surfaces.

Laser protective eyewear is a well-recognized precaution and includes wrap around glasses and goggles which are rated by optical density at various wavelengths. An optical density of more than 4 at the particular wavelength of laser used is considered safe for dermatologic lasers. The laser operator, assistants, and patients should wear protective goggles while the laser is in operation. Glass eye wears are heavy, reflect light, and the protective coating may get scratched. Plastic goggles on the other hand are lightweight, absorb light, but can crack or melt at high temperatures. Once again, it cannot be overemphasized that each set of goggles should have specific wavelength of rejection which should match the emission spectrum of the specific laser in use.[4]

Patients should be made to wear eye shields covering the eyes, thus protecting the entire periorbital area. These eye shields can be used while the laser is performed away from the eyes. When the laser is performed near the periorbital area, corneal shields are preferred. Heat proof stainless steel corneal shields are used as they reflect the light and do not crack like plastic eye shields. Proparacaine hydrochloride anesthetic eye drops are instilled to the cornea before insertion of the corneal shields.

❑ EYE CARE DURING FILLERS[5]

Key Prevention Strategies

- Know the location and depth of facial vessels and the common variations. Injectors should understand the appropriate depth and plane of injection at different sites

- Inject slowly and with minimal pressure
- Inject in small increments so that any filler injected into the artery can be flushed peripherally before the next incremental injection. This prevents the column of filler traveling retrograde. No more than 0.1 mL of filler should be injected with each increment
- Move the needle tip while injecting, so as not to deliver a large deposit in one location
- Aspirate before injection. This recommendation is controversial as it may not be possible to get flash back in to a syringe through fine needles with thick gels. In addition, the small size and collapsibility of facial vessels limit the efficacy
- Use a small diameter needle. A smaller needle necessitates slower injection and is less likely to occlude the vessel
- Smaller syringes are preferred to larger once as a large syringe may make it more challenging to control the volume and increases the probability of injecting a larger bolus
- Consider using a cannula, as they are less likely to pierce a blood vessel. Some authors recommended use of the cannula in the medical cheek, tear trough, and nasolabial fold in particular
- Use extreme caution when injecting a patient who undergone previous surgical procedure in the area
- Consider missing the pillar with epinephrine to promote vasoconstriction as cannulating a vasoconstricted artery is more difficult.

Key Management Strategies

- If a patient complains of ocular pain or vision changes, stop the injection at once. Immediately contact an ophthalmologist or oculoplastic colleague and urgently transfer the patient directly there

- Consider treating the injected area and surrounding location with hyaluronidase if hyaluronic acid filler is used
- Consider retrobulbar injection of 300–600 units (2–4 mL) of hyaluronidase if hyaluronic acid filler is used
- Reduction of intraocular pressure should be considered. Mechanisms to achieve this include ocular massage, anterior chamber paracentesis, intravenous mannitol, and acetazolamide
- Given the relatively high prevalence of central nervous system complications that accompany blindness, it is important to monitor the patient's neurologic status and consider ordering imaging studies of the brain if visual complications occur.

❑ CONCLUSION

Ocular injury during laser therapy is uncommon. Direct laser light injury can cause burns and vision loss. Vascular lasers and Q switched Nd YAG laser destroy retinal vasculature, while iris atrophy occurs in IPL exposure. Late complication is nuclear cataract. Ablative lasers rapidly injure the cornea.

Almost all laser eye injury is preventable with the use of eye shields for patients and appropriate laser goggles for the operator.

❑ REFERENCES

1. Barkhana Y, Belkin M. Laser eye injuries: Surv Ophthalmol. 2000;44:459-78.
2. Friedman NR, Saleeby ER, Rubin MG, Sander T, Krull CA. Safety parameters for avoiding acute ocular damage from the reflected CO_2 (10.6 μm) laser beam. J Am Acad Dermatol. 1987;17:815-8.
3. Cao LY, Taylor JS, Vidimos A. Patient safety in dermatology: a review of the literature. Dermatol Online J. 2010;16:3.
4. Lolis Margarita, Dunbar SW, Goldberg DJ, Hansen TJ, MacFarlane DF. Patient safety in procedural dermatology. J Am Acad Dermatol. 2015;73(1):15-24.

Managing Medical Emergencies in the Office: Office Emergency

Prashant Mallya

❏ INTRODUCTION

Medical emergencies can occur any time.[1] The best way to handle an emergency is to be prepared in advance. All office staff should be prepared to recognize and handle medical emergencies. This chapter provides guidance and recommendation concerning common medical emergencies in the office. It describes assessment of patient, resuscitation procedures and equipment, and use of emergency drugs in office practice.

❏ OVERVIEW

Medical emergency can occur unexpectedly and can lead to medical crises. The type of medical emergency that occur in office setup are vast some include:

- Asthmatic attack
- Myocardial infraction
- Sudden cardiac death
- Hypoglycemia
- Allergic reaction.

In an office setup, medical emergencies might be directly related to treatment or procedure or may occur by chance.[2] For example, a patient waiting for a procedure may have a sudden cardiac death or a patient might experience an allergic reaction during a procedure.

To manage these emergencies, one must be aware how to prevent this circumstance and how to appropriately respond if an emergency situation does arise.

❏ PREVENTION

Knowing your patient is an important step in preventing emergencies. Never perform procedure on strangers, this can be done by proper history taking and physical examination.[3] Physical examination will not only give the baseline vitals of the patient but will also help in monitoring the patient's condition during and after the procedure. History and physical examination of a patient can help to proactively access the patient's risk of a medical emergency.

❏ STAFF ROLES AND RESPONSIBILITIES

One of the first steps in designing an emergency response plan is to assign staff roles and responsibilities, "offices should use all to their staff effectively and have a proactive team approach."[4] The approach should reinforce the important role that each staff member plays in emergency preparedness, and it should stress that appropriate preparation can potentially improve patient's outcome.[5]

The size of the practice and staff member's skill and training will help shape specific roles and responsibilities.

❏ CLASSIFICATION OF OFFICE PROCEDURES

The term levels 1–3 rulers to complexity of surgeries.

Level 1

Minor surgical procedure such as excision of skin lesion, performed under topical or local anesthetic and not involving drug induced alteration of consciousness other than minimal sedation utilizing preoperative oral anxiolytic medication.

Level 2

Minor or major surgical procedure in conjunction with oral, parental or intravenous sedation or under analgesic or dissociative drugs.

Level 3

Surgical procedures that require deep sedation, analgesic, general anesthetic, or major conduction block and support of vital bodily functions.[6]

Office based setting providing level 3 and probably level 2 type or surgeries should maintain current advanced cardiac like support (ACLS) certification. At least one assistant should have current certification in ACLS and other assistant should maintain training in

basic cardiopulmonary resuscitation (basic life support). This requirement can vary from place to place.

❏ MANAGING EMERGENCIES

Managing emergencies is a team effort, staff members should be trained to monitor and interpret vital signs. All staff member should be trained in basic life support. The office should also have a written emergency protocol and emergency phone numbers (nearby hospital, ambulance) pasted on the wall. Apart from all these, every office where different level of procedures are carried out must be equipped with emergency equipment's and drugs.[7]

Emergency Medical Equipment

- Anesthestic machine (in level 3 procedures)
- Oxygen Ambu bag, mask, oxygen cylinder
- Disposable syringes
- Intravenous cannulas and intravenous sets
- Intravenous fluids (normal saline, dextrose)
- Sphygmomanometer meter/stethoscope
- Pulse oximeter for monitoring vitals
- Suction apparatus and suction catheter
- Glucometer
- Defibrillator.

Emergency Drugs

- Adrenaline (epinephrine) 1:1,000 (1 mg/cc)
- Atropine ampules
- Diazepam for convulsion
- Dopamin ampule
- Hydrocortisone, 100 mg vial (powder form)
- Nitroglycerine ampule
- Pheniramine ampule (antihistamine)
- 50% dextrose for ondansetron.

Emergency equipment and medicines should be stored in a designated location and accessible at all time. Emergency kit should be labeled and easy to transport.

❑ RECOGNITION OF AN EMERGENCY AND INITIAL EMERGENCY PROCEDURE

When an emergency situation is recognized, procedure should be immediately stopped and summoned for help. Establish patient responsiveness by shaking or asking with loud voice (are you okay?), lay the patient in supine position, check for presence of carotid pulse not more than 5–10 seconds. If no pulse is presented, start cardiopulmonary resuscitation (CPR) (Figures 1 and 2).

The 2010 American Heart Association guidelines for cardiopulmonary resuscitation C-A-B (chest compression, airway and breathiness) consider definitive treatment, drugs only after following C-A-B sequence (Flowchart 1).

❑ SAMPLE EMERGENCY ASSIGNMENTS

Receptionist
- Call emergency numbers
- Calm persons in reception area
- Direct reserve squad to patients.

Assistant 1
- Maintain C-A-B of CPR
- Assess and record vital signs.

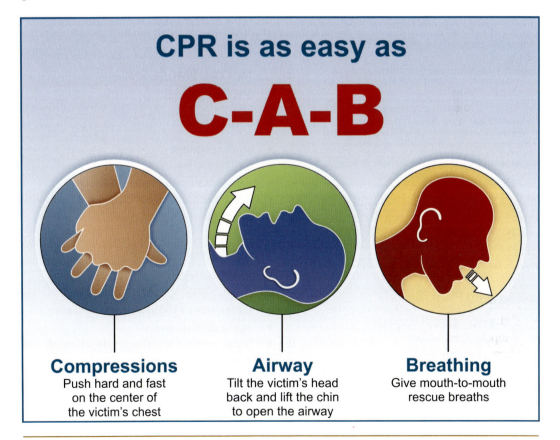

Figure 1: Steps of cardiopulmonary resuscitation.

CPR, cardiopulmonary resuscitation.

Chest compressions come first now
New cardiopulmonary resuscitation guidelines show the importance of starting chest compressions immediately, instead of opening the victim's airway and breathing into their mouth first

Cardiopulmonary resuscitation revised guidelines: Think C-A-B

Compressions	**Airway**	**Breathing**
Push at least 2 inches on adult breastbone, 100 times per minute, to move oxygenated blood to vital organs	Open the airway and check for breathing or blockage; watch for rise of chest, and listen for air movement	Tilt chin back for the unobstructed passing of air; give two breaths, and resume chest compressions

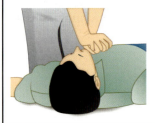 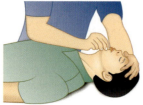 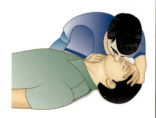

Figure 2: New revised guidlines of cardiopulmonary resuscitation

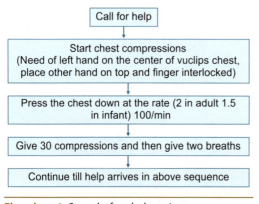

```
Call for help
     ↓
Start chest compressions
(Need of left hand on the center of vuclips chest,
place other hand on top and finger interlocked)
     ↓
Press the chest down at the rate (2 in adult 1.5
in infant) 100/min
     ↓
Give 30 compressions and then give two breaths
     ↓
Continue till help arrives in above sequence
```

Flowchart 1: Steps before help arrives.

Assistant 2

- Bring emergency kit/oxygen
- Prepare medications
- Turns to appropriate page in emergency reference.

Consultant

- Directs team member and overall treatment
- Administer emergency medication.

❑ INITIAL EMERGENCY PROCEDURE

Recognization

- Stop treatment
- Call for help
- Assess consciousness, if unconscious
- Raise the leg above with patient in supine position.

Assess Circulation

- Check for pulse
- If no pulse, begin chest compression (at the rate of 100/min 30 compression)
- Apply defibrillator
- If pulse present, check rate, then assess airway.

Access of Airway

- Use head-tilt/chin-lift, this way airway is opened
- Suction the throat if necessary.

Assess Breathing

- Check for breathing
- If not, give two rescue breath with pocket mask and continue CPR
- Call for defibrillator.

Assess Patient and Situation

- Manage situation as appropriate to diagnose
- Take and record vital signs to patient breathing with pulse
- Never attempt to transport patient yourself
- Call ambulance
- Cardiac arrest
- Respiratory arrest
- Chest pain/seizure
- Unconsciousness
- Treat patient supportively till rescue help arrives
- Fill out office medical emergency report.

❑ ALLERGY/ANAPHYLAXIS

An allergic reaction is the result of an antigen-antibody reaction to a substance which the patient has been previously sensitized. This could be triggered by, antibiotics, local anesthetics, latex, or nonsteroidal anti-inflammatory drugs.

Signs of Anaphylaxis

- Red rashes, hives
- Swollen throat and lips
- Wheezing
- Hoarse voice
- Trouble in swallowing
- Vomiting
- Chest tightness
- Pale color on face.

Management of Anaphylaxes

- Remove the trigger
- Assess and maintain circulation airway and breathing

- Call for help, connect the monitor
- Inject adrenaline 1:1,000–0.5 mg slc or intramuscular mid-thigh can repeat in 5–15 minutes if needed
- Place the patient on the back and elevate the lower extremities
- High flow oxygen supplementation
- Establish intravenous access using wide bore cannula, if hypotension 20 mg/kg of 0.9% saline rapidly
- Inject hydrocortisone 100 mg intravenously
- Inject diphenhydramine intravenously
- If patient has cardiac arrest, then CPR has to be performed.

❑ CONCLUSION

Emergencies in an office procedure can occur before the procedure due to patient's preexisting medical illness; can also occur during the procedure such as allergic reactions to injections and anaphylaxis, vasovagal attack etc.

Medical emergencies can occur during office procedures. Managed properly, most emergencies are resolved satisfactorily 95% of life threatening situations can be prevented and 5% will occur in spite of all preventive efforts.

❑ REFERENCES

1. Toback SL. Medical emergency preparedness in office practice. Am Fam Physician. 2007;75(11):1679-84.
2. Rosenberg M. Preparing for medical emergencies. The essential drugs and equipment for dental office. J Am Dent Assoc. 2010;141(Suppl 1)145-95.
3. Malamed SF. Knowing your patient. J Am Den Assoc. 2010;141 Suppl 1:3S-7S.
4. Scmpowski IP, Brison RJ. Dealing with office emergencies stepwise approach for family medicine. Can Fam Physician. 2002;48:1464-72.
5. Hass DA. Preparing dental office staff members or emergencies developing basic action plans. J Am Dent Assoc. 2010;141(Suppl 1):85-135.
6. Twersky RS, Philip BK, editors. Handbook of ambulatory anesthesia. 2nd ed. New York: Springer; 2008.
7. Rosenberg, Preparing for medical emergencies; ADA council on scientific affairs, office emergencies and emergency icets; Toback medical emergency preparedness, Scpowski, Dealing with office emergencies.

Suturing for Dermatologists

Kuldeep Singh

❑ INTRODUCTION

Learning suturing skills is an important need for the modern dermatologist. Whether it is a minor surgical procedure like a biopsy from the face , or a laceration one may be required to repair surgically, the ability to provide a fine scar goes a long way. The endeavor has been to filter out unnecessary information, and provide clear, relevant, and workable knowledge to the reader.

❑ OBJECTIVE OF SUTURING

The objective of suturing is to obtain gentle closure of healthy skin edges, healing and restoration of tensile strength of the wound. Suturing is defined as uniting of two edges with sutures.[1] It is a very simple concept, but good suturing requires a high level of concentration, understanding of the concept of wound healing, knowledge of suture materials, and wound behavior with regards to healing and scar formation.[2]

❑ INDICATIONS FOR DERMATOLOGISTS

Dermatologists will need to utilize principles and skills of suturing for:

- Excision biopsies
- Excision of small lesions
- Emergency repair of small lacerations (if a surgeon is not available)
- Miscellaneous.

❑ MATERIALS AVAILABLE

Suturing materials as well as needles have undergone modifications many times in the last 3 decades. Eyeless or atraumatic needles are the norm now. These needles are hollow at the rear end and the suture is swaged into the hollow rear of the needle. The purpose was to prevent the rear end of the needle making a larger hole in the tissues than the tip of the needle.

Needles come with variations in curvature and design of the tip. Commonly, curved needles are 3/8 of a circle, but half circle and 5/8 (more than half circle) curvature are also available (Figure 1). The 5/8 circle needle is not suitable for skin suturing for dermatologists and should be avoided.

The tip of the needle comes as either a cutting tip (leading edge is sharp-best used for suturing the skin), but a reverse cutting tip (trailing edge is sharp) comes with finer sutures to minimize enlarging the hole in the skin as

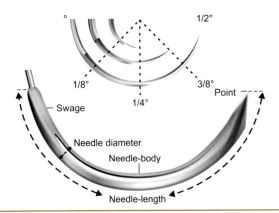

Figure 1: Needle anatomy

we drag the needle out, or a round body tip (smooth tip) which is completely atraumatic, but is not suitable for suturing of the skin, and must be avoided. (Figures 2 to 4).

Needle length and diameter are also variable, but usually, this is prefixed according to thickness (diameter) of the suture.

Sutures come in various sizes starting from number 2 to 11-0 (USP). As the number goes on increasing from 1-0 to 11-0 the suture keeps getting thinner in diameter with 11-0 the thinnest. Sutures for practical use for dermatologists range from 4-0 to 6-0.

Suture material is available in 2 variations—absorbable and nonabsorbable. Absorbable sutures are mainly used as buried sutures (muscle layer, subcutaneous, or dermal) and do not need to be removed, while nonabsorbable sutures are used on the skin surface, and have to be removed.

Absorbable suture most commonly used is polyglactin 910 (Vicryl) which is an absorbable braided suture. It is dyed violet in color, but undyed version is also available. It handles and knots well and is degraded by hydrolysis. Only 25% tensile strength remains at 4 weeks, although suture remains for up to 70 days. Buried subcuticular PDS II (polydioxanone) gave better scars in terms of appearance in a study by Alam et al.[3]

Poliglecaprone (Monocryl) is an absorbable undyed monofilament suture. It is also degraded by hydrolysis. It is easy to handle and knot, but has poor visualization due to its uncolored nature. It lasts long enough for healing with 30–40% tensile strength remaining at 2 weeks, suture absorption happening by 119 days.

Polydioxanone (PDS II) is a monofilament absorbable suture, dyed blue, is difficult to handle, as well as knot, but remains the longest lasting absorbable suture compared to Monocryl and Vicryl, with 60% residual tensile strength at 4 weeks, and stays for about 238 days. It is available with a round bodied needle tip as well as a cutting tip needle, therefore, dermal suturing is easy with this suture also.

Nylon (Ethilon) is the most commonly used nonabsorbable suture. It is available in all sizes and is dyed black in color and is a monofilament strand. It is available with a cutting needle and therefore suitable for suturing the skin.

Polypropylene (Prolene) is a monofilament nonabsorbable suture and is blue in color. The knotting ease is less than nylon, and it has a strong memory and tends to assume the shape it has when packed.

Silk (no one uses it now) sutures are made from silk fibers extracted from the silkworm

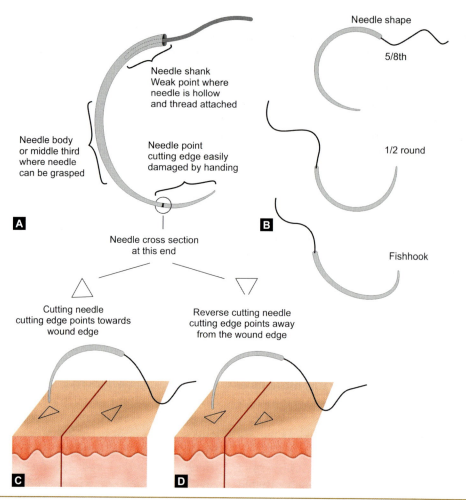

Figure 2: Showing **A,** different parts of the needle and **B,** various types of needles according to curvature and tip profile (right), **C,** 3/8 circle needles showing the leading edge sharp (cutting needle) and **D,** trailing edge sharp (reverse cutting–bottom right)

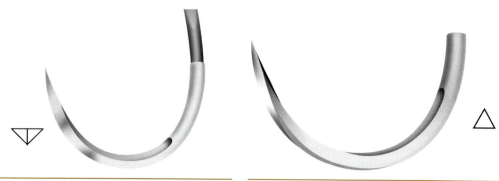

Figure 3: Cutting needle tip—outside edge (leading) sharp

Figure 4: Reverse cutting needle tip—inside (trailing) edge sharp

Bombyx mori. They are braided (polyfilament), coated, dyed black, and are nonabsorbable. This suture shows maximum ease of handling and knot tying, but tensile strength is not very high. Silk invokes an inflammatory reaction if left long enough in tissues, likely to produce more scarring.

The advantage of nonabsorbable monofilament sutures (nylon and prolene) is that they slip easily through tissues, and can be left in longer without risking additional scarring. The flip side is that they are difficult to handle or knot easily. The braided sutures on the other hand are easy to handle and tie, but have a greater drag, and by the wicking action more likely to harbor bacteria.

❑ BASICS OF WOUND HEALING

All wounds including surgical wounds heal with scarring. Initially, there is an inflammatory phase with outpouring of edema fluid and neutrophils, followed by the proliferative phase with presence of macrophages and fibroblasts. The suture line gains 3–5% tensile strength by 2 weeks, 20% by 3 weeks, and 50% by one month.[4]

Scars tend to stretch apart till 9 weeks from suturing as they are subject to elastic pull of the skin, as well as external forces of muscle contraction and movements. About 80% of tensile strength is gained at 9 weeks.[5] Therefore, scars on the moving parts, i.e., extremities, scars placed at 90° to the skin creases (relaxed skin tension lines), or where there is excessive tension on the suture line to begin with, tend to stretch wider than those on the face, along skin creases and those with no tension on the suture line to begin with, or where deeper suture layer has taken away skin tension.

Needle holders: today, all suturing as well as knot tying is done with needle holders, and not with hands. A needle holder consists of a grip, a ratchet or lock, a shank, hinge and jaws/tip. A 6 inches long needle holder (Mayo needle holder—Figure 5) with a ratchet, with a short, narrow beak with a tungsten carbide tip (Golden Handle) is good to suture superficial incisions/wounds. The Olsen Hegar needle holder (Figure 6) has a scissors incorporated in the proximal part of the jaws to cut suture, and is extremely helpful when suturing alone.

The needle is held a little behind the tip of the needle holder, perpendicular to the jaws, a little behind the middle of the needle (Figure 7) using the thumb and the ring finger, with the index finger resting on the shank to stabilize the needle holder (Figure 8). A fine toothed Adson forceps is a good companion to hold skin edges while suturing. Contrary to perception, nontoothed forceps is more traumatic, and should be used only for suture removal (Figures 9 and 10).

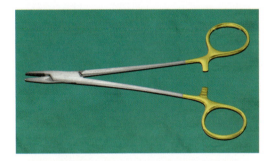

Figure 5: Mayo needle holder 6 inches with tungsten carbide tip.

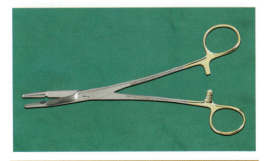

Figure 6: Olsen Hegar needle holder 6.5 inches with scissors tungsten carbide tip.

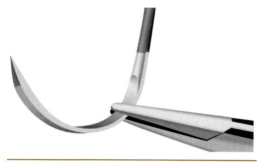

Figure 7: Technique of holding the needle in the jaws of the needle holder. Grasp the needle one-third of the distance from the swaged end to the point

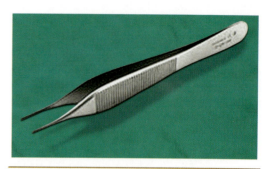

Figure 9: Nontoothed Adson forceps (for suture removal).

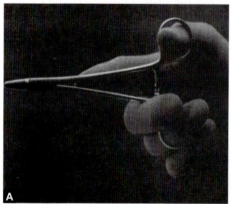

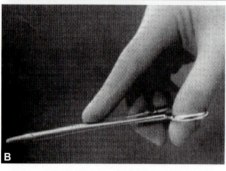

Figure 8: Technique of holding needle holder— thumb and middle or ring fingers inside the finger rings, with the index finger stabilizing the shank.

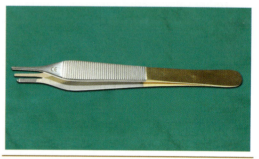

Figure 10: Toothed Adson forceps (ideal for holding tissues during suturing).

❑ SUTURING TECHNIQUES

The most useful suturing technique is the one which everts the edges slightly to achieve good edge to edge approximation, is snug, not tight, has minimal or an external pull on the suture line, and suture remains strong for at least 6 weeks.

Simple interrupted skin suture is the most commonly used. The key element is to achieve uniform contact of incision/wound edges from bottom to the top with mild eversion of edges and with just enough tension to snugly hold them together and not be tight. The wrist is pronated completely to allow needle to enter the skin at an angle of 90°. Gather a wider bite of tissue in the depth (Figure 11) compared to that on the surface. The knot should be tied on one side of the wound rather than in the center, as it will facilitate heaping up of the edges to cause mild eversion. There should be no blanching of the skin lying within the suture, indicating excessive tightening of suture and then it must be loosened or reapplied.

The vertical mattress suture is used when the skin edges tend to invert while applying a suture. The technique is shown in figure 12. If one has applied good deeper sutures, the skin suture will not tend to invert, and a mattress suture is not required. Remember, 2 holes are

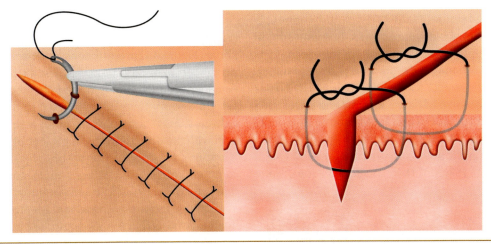

Figure 11: Simple interrupted suture—needle should enter at an angle of 90° to the skin surface.

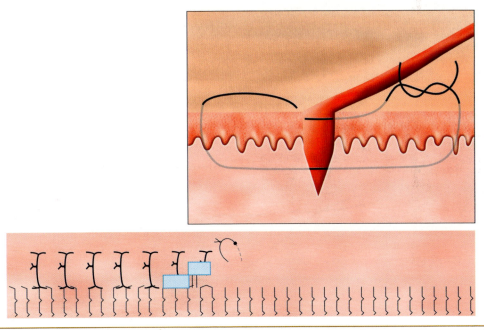

Figure 12: Vertical mattress suture—first needle punctures away-away, second punctures near-near to skin edge, then secured with a square knot.

better than 4 in terms of minimizing the scar, so these are best avoided on the face. Also, the mattress suture when tied tends to easily produce more tension on the suture line and assessment of correct skin tension is difficult.

The continuous subcuticular (dermal) buried suture (Figure 13) is a suture commonly used to avoid suture marks. But, one should remember that amount of scar formed is proportional to the amount of dermal injury. This is mainly used to approximate the outer layer of skin of long incisions, and never used for traumatic wounds. Monocryl is usually used and both ends are tied deep and buried.[6]

Continuous subcuticular pull through suture (Figure 14): in smaller incisions, some

people use continuous subcuticular nylon or prolene sutures. These are kept untied at the ends and projecting out, so that they can be removed after healing, by pulling at either end. They are usually removed at 7–21 days depending on the duration of support needed.

Knotting techniques: the square knot (Figure 15), the half hitch, and the surgeons knots (Figure 16) are the ones one needs to master. In skin suturing, the first throw is usually not straight but a half hitch, with the second throw square, adjusting to the correct tightness, and then converted into a square knot with the third throw to lock it (Figure 17). If there is tension on the tissue edges, the surgeons knot is used with a double straight throw, followed by a single straight throw, and another one locking it. The advantage of a first double throw is that it does not loosen as you are taking the second throw. Also, if you do not have an assistant to hold the knot, the first double throw will do the trick.

The dermal sutures should have their knots tied deep, and are also called inverted sutures. Taking a bite through the dermis in your

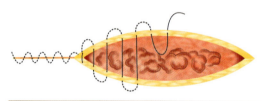

Figure 13: Continuous buried dermal (subcuticular) suture.

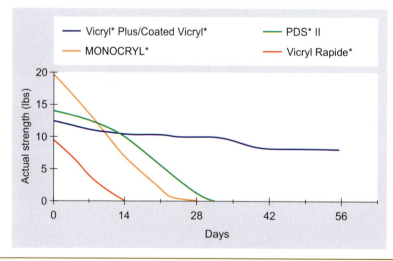

Figure 14: Tensile strength loss with time for various absorbable sutures—longest for PDS II (polydioxanone).

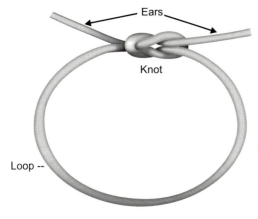

Figure 15: Square knot—first throw is single and the ears (ends of sutures) cross over to the opposite side. Second throw is in reverse direction squaring the knot (locking it).

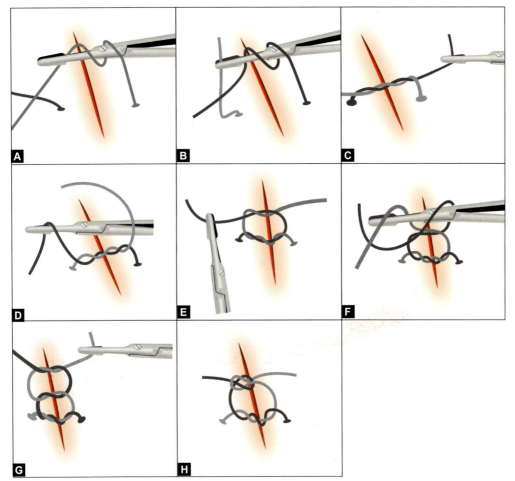

Figure 16: Technique of tying a surgeons knot: **A–C,** first double throw being tied-note crossing over of suture to opposite sides; **D** and **E,** Second throw single-again crossing over of suture ends to the other side. **F–H,** A third throw making the second knot square and locking it.

deeper stitch holds the skin edges together, and reduces tension on the skin sutures. Also, as the skin sutures are removed early, to minimize scarring, a long-acting dermal suture will prevent the scar from stretching by offering prolonged dermal support (Figure 18).

Suture removal: suture lines are kept clean and free of crust till the time they need to be removed. This is achieved by either protecting it by a dressing, which is changed at regular intervals, or by cleaning the crusts. Sutures are removed from the eyelids in 5 days, face in 7 days, body in 10 days, and hands and feet in 10–14 days. There is no evidence of a difference in scar using different suture materials, if sutures are removed within 7 days.

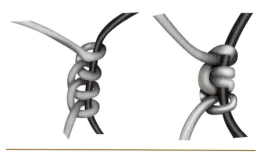

Figure 17: The half hitch knot A, with multiple half hitch throws. Notice each throw is not crossing over to the other side like in a square throw. It can still loosen the knot. The locked half-half hitch knot B, is done by making the next throw straight like in a square knot and locking it securely.

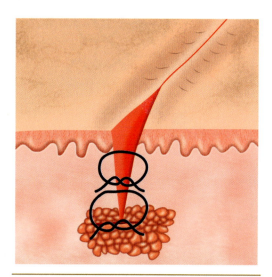

Figure 18: Dead space left in the middle should be obliterated by another suture. Also showing the inverted dermal suture with the knot tied deep.

❑ CONCLUSION

Incisions should be planned in skin creases wherever possible, otherwise parallel to them or as close to parallel. Tension can be reduced on the skin repair by good deeper tissue approximation. Visible scars from suture marks arise only if the suture is tight, or there is tension on the skin edges. Simple interrupted sutures are better than mattress sutures. Needle should be held a little behind the middle of the needle using a needle holder. The tip of the needle should be grasped a little behind the tip while retrieving it, to avoid blunting the tip.[7] The entry angle of needle into skin should be 90° to prevent inversion of edges. Round bodied needle cannot pierce skin, hence, use cutting, taper cut, or reverse cutting needles. Do not use absorbable suture on the skin as interrupted sutures. One can use them as either interrupted or continuous buried dermal absorbable suture. Skin sutures should be removed by the day 7 on the face, by 10 days on the trunk, and by 14 days on the lower limbs. Using PDS II for prolonged dermal support as interrupted dermal sutures, where more tension is anticipated, gives a less wider scar.[8] External support with Steri-Strips will minimize stretching of scar, if used for at least 6–8 weeks after suture removal.[9,10]

❑ REFERENCES

1. Stedman's medical dictionary. 23rd ed. Philadelphia: Williams & Wilkins; 1976.

2. Odland PB, Muragami CS. Simple suture techniques and knot tying. In: Wheeland RG, (Ed). Cutaneous surgery. Philadelphia: Saunders; 1984. p. 178.

3. Alam M, Posten W, Martini MC, Wrone DA, Rademaker AW. Aesthetic and functional efficacy of subcuticular running epidermal closures of the trunk and extremity: a rater-blinded randomized control trial. Arch Dermatol. 2006;142(10):1272-8.

4. Kudur MH, Pai SB, Sripathi H, Prabhu S. Sutures and suturing techniques in skin closure. Indian J Dermatol Venereol Leprol. 2009;75:425-34.

5. Goslen JB. Wound healing for the dermatologic surgeon. J Dermatol Surg Oncol. 1998;14:959-72.

6. Farquharson M, Hollingshead J, Moran B. Surgery of the skin and subcutaneous tissue. In: Farquharson's textbook of operative general surgery. 10th ed. Roca Baton: CRC Press; 2014. p. 17.

7. Holt GR, Holt JE. Suture materials and technique. Ear Nose Throat J. 1981;60:12.

8. Elliot D, Mahaffey PJ. The stretched scar: the benefit of prolonged dermal support. Br J Plast Surg. 1989;42(1): 74-8.

9. Kia KF, Burns MV, Vandergriff T, Weitzul S. Prevention of scar spread on trunk excisions: a rater-blinded randomized controlled trial. JAMA Dermatol. 2013;149(6):687-91.

10. Rosengren H, Askew DA, Heal C, Buettner PG, Humphreys WO, Semmens LA. Does taping torso scars following dermatologic surgery improve scar appearance? Dermatol Pract Concept. 2013;3(2):75-83

Index

Page numbers followed by *f* refer to figure, *t* refer to table, and *b* refer to box.